1
Low Carb & No Cookbook. (A) 130- (B) 85-Low Carb Des 27-Restaurant Guide To Eating Out.

LOW CARB & NO CARB COOKBOOK
130 RECIPES

****
****

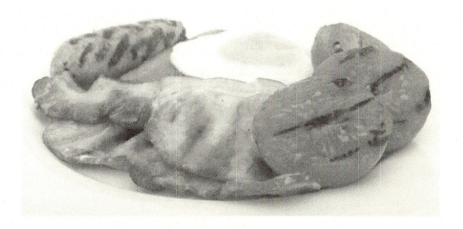

BREAKFAST

2
Low Carb & No Carb Cookbook. (A) 130-Recipes. (B) 85-Low Carb Desserts. (C) 27-Restaurant Guide To Eating Out.

(1) <u>**CRUSTLESS QUICHE - 4 Servings**</u>

1/2 cup heavy cream (4.8 g carbs) 1/2 cup water
1/4 cup green onions (1.7 g)
8 whole eggs
2 cups crumbled bacon (cooked & cooled) 1 cup shredded cheese
1/2 cup fresh or frozen spinach (1.2 g)

Preheat oven 350 degrees. Beat eggs. Fold in remaining ingredients. Pour into glass casserole dish (sprayed with cooking oil). Bake for 45 minutes-1 hour.

Carb Count: Recipe Total 7.7 g, Per Serving 1.9 g

(2) <u>**MOCK FRENCH TOAST - 4 Servings**</u>

6 ounces unflavored pork rinds
4 eggs

3
Low Carb & No Carb Cookbook. (A) 130-Recipes. (B) 85-Low Carb Desserts. (C) 27-Restaurant Guide To Eating Out.

1/2 cup heavy cream (4.8 g)
6 packets artificial sweetener
1 tsp cinnamon (1.8 g)
1 tsp vanilla extract

Crumble pork rinds up until they resemble bread crumbs and set aside. Beat eggs. Add remaining ingredients and mix well. Add crushed pork rinds to the egg mixture and allow to sit for approximately 5 minutes. Meanwhile, heat butter or oil in a skillet. Pour onto skillet 1/8 cup at a time. Heat, turning once. Serve with blackberry syrup, maple butter or low carb maple syrup (Recipes #28-30).

Carb Count: Recipe Total 6.6 g, Per Serving 1.6 g

(3) <u>LOW CARB WAFFLES - 6 Servings</u>

4

l
a
r
g
e

e
g
g
s
,

s
e

4
Low Carb & No Carb Cookbook. (A) 130-Recipes. (B) 85-Low Carb Desserts. (C) 27-Restaurant Guide To Eating Out.

separated

4 tbsp butter

1/4 cup oat flour (8 g)
3/4 cup sour cream (12 g)
1/2 tsp vanilla extract
1/2 tsp salt

Beat the egg whites with an electric mixer until they form soft peaks. Set aside. In another bowl, cream the butter until fluffy and beat in the egg yolks one at a time. Add the oat flour and sour cream and mix well. Add a little water, if needed, to reach desired consistency. Stir in the vanilla and salt. Fold in the egg whites. Bake in a preheated waffle iron. Serve with

5
Low Carb & No Carb Cookbook. (A) 130-Recipes. (B) 85-Low Carb Desserts. (C) 27-Restaurant Guide To Eating Out.

blackberry syrup, maple butter or low carb maple syrup (Recipes #28-30).

Carb Count: Recipe Total 20 g, Per Serving: 3.3 g

(4) <u>ZUCCHINI HASH BROWNS - 4 servings</u>

butter
2 cups shredded zucchini (7.7 g)
1/4 tsp salt
2 eggs
4 tbsp Parmesan cheese

Combine zucchini with salt. Let stand for 15 minutes. Absorb excess moisture with paper towels. Combine zucchini with eggs and cheese. Make small flat patties with batter. Melt butter in a skillet. Cook patties, turning once, until golden on both sides.

Carb Count: Recipe Total 7.7 g, Per Serving: 1.9 g

(5) <u>BACON CHEESE MUFFINS - 6 Servings</u>

1 cup high gluten flour (24 g)
3

t
s
p

b
a
k
i

6
Low Carb & No Carb Cookbook. (A) 130-Recipes. (B) 85-Low Carb Desserts. (C) 27-Restaurant Guide To Eating Out.

ng powder

1/4 tsp salt

1/2 cup cream

7
Low Carb & No Carb Cookbook. (A) 130-Recipes. (B) 85-Low Carb Desserts. (C) 27-Restaurant Guide To Eating Out.

(4.8g) 1/2 cup water 4 eggs, beaten

8
Low Carb & No Carb Cookbook. (A) 130-Recipes. (B) 85-Low Carb Desserts. (C) 27-Restaurant Guide To Eating Out.

shredded cheese

16 slices bacon, cooked & crumbled

Preheat oven to 400 degrees. Combine flour, baking powder & salt. In a separate bowl, combine cream, water & eggs. Mix wet & dry ingredients. Stir in shredded cheese & bacon. Pour into muffin tin. Bake for 20 minutes.

Carb Count: Recipe Total: 28.8 g, Per Serving: 4.8 g

(6) CHEESE BLINTZES - 2 Servings

4 egg whites
3/4 cup cottage cheese (4.5 g)
1/2 cup strawberries (5.2 g)
4 tbsp sour cream (2 g)

Combine egg whites & cottage cheese. Lightly spray nonstick skillet. Heat over

9
Low Carb & No Carb Cookbook. (A) 130-Recipes. (B) 85-Low Carb Desserts. (C) 27-Restaurant Guide To Eating Out.

medium heat. Using half of the batter, cook for a few minutes on each side. Repeat with remaining batter. Serve with fruit & sour cream.

Carb Count: Recipe Total: 11.7 g, Per Serving: 5.8 g

(7) COTTAGE SCRAMBLED EGGS - 4 Servings

6 whole eggs
1/4 cup cream (2.4 g)
1/4 cup water
1/2 tsp sa

10
Low Carb & No Carb Cookbook. (A) 130-Recipes. (B) 85-Low Carb Desserts. (C) 27-Restaurant Guide To Eating Out.

1 t

1/4 tsp pepper
1 cup cottage cheese (6 g) 3 tbsp

11
Low Carb & No Carb Cookbook. (A) 130-Recipes. (B) 85-Low Carb Desserts. (C) 27-Restaurant Guide To Eating Out.

butter
1 tomato sliced (5.8 g)

Beat eggs with cream, water, salt and pepper. Fold in cottage cheese.
Heat butter in skillet & cook egg mixture in skillet. Serve with tomato.
Carb Count: Recipe Total 14.2 g, Per Serving: 3.7 g

(8) APPLE & BRIE EGGS - 4 Servings

1 small apple; peeled, cored & chopped (10 g)
Butter
8 eggs
1/4 cup light cream (1.2 g)
salt & pe

12
Low Carb & No Carb Cookbook. (A) 130-Recipes. (B) 85-Low Carb Desserts. (C) 27-Restaurant Guide To Eating Out.

pp
er
1/2 cup crumbled Brie cheese

Melt butter in skillet. Sauté apple in butter. Beat together eggs, cream, salt & pepper. Melt butter in pan. Pour in egg mixture and scramble. Add apples & brie. Warm & serve.

Carb Count: Recipe Total 11.2 g, Per Serving: 2.8 g

(9) <u>LOW CARB PANCAKES - 2 Servings</u>

1/3 cup milk & egg protein powder
1/3 cup ricotta cheese (2.3 g)
2

t
b
s
p

h
e
a
v
y
c
r
e
a
m

(
1

13

Low Carb & No Carb Cookbook. (A) 130-Recipes. (B) 85-Low Carb Desserts. (C) 27-Restaurant Guide To Eating Out.

.2 g) 1 tbsp water 2 packets artificial sweetener 1 egg 1/4 ts

14
Low Carb & No Carb Cookbook. (A) 130-Recipes. (B) 85-Low Carb Desserts. (C) 27-Restaurant Guide To Eating Out.

p baking powder 1/8 tsp cinnamon (0.2

15
Low Carb & No Carb Cookbook. (A) 130-Recipes. (B) 85-Low Carb Desserts. (C) 27-Restaurant Guide To Eating Out.

g
)

pinch nutmeg

Blend all ingredients until smooth. Cook on medium-low heat; turn carefully when edges are set and bubbly throughout. Serve with butter and low carb syrup. Enjoy!

Carb Count: Recipe Total 3.7 g, Per Serving 1.8 g

(10) FRITTATA - 2 Servings

1/4 cup cauliflower (1.5 g)
1/4 cup shredded zucchini (0.8 g)
3 whole eggs
4 ounces deli ham, sliced & chopped
1 cup shredded cheese
salt & pepper

Preheat oven to 375 degrees. Heat oil in pan. Add cauliflower & zucchini to skillet & cook 5-6 minutes, stirring occasionally. Beat the eggs. Remove vegetables from skillet & add to eggs. Pour in glass dish (sprayed with oil), add ham & cheese and bake for 30-35 minutes or until cooked thoroughly.

Carb Count: Recipe Total 5 g, Per Serving 2.5 g

(11) SOUTHWEST QUICHE

8 whole eggs
1/2 cup heavy cream (4.8 g carbs) 1/2 cup water
1/4 cup green onions (1.7 g)
1 tbsp chili powder (4 g) 1 tsp cumin (0.9 g)
2 cups cooked chicken, cut in bite sized pieces
1 cup shredded cheese
1/2 cup fresh or frozen spinach (1.2 g)

Preheat oven 350 degrees. Beat eggs. Fold in remaining ingredients. Pour into glass casserole dish (sprayed with cooking oil). Bake for 45 minutes-1 hour.

Carb Count: Recipe Total 12.6 g, Per Serving 3.2 g

(12) BACON BREAKFAST PIE - 2 Servings

1/2 cup shredded cheese

17

Low Carb & No Carb Cookbook. (A) 130-Recipes. (B) 85-Low Carb Desserts. (C) 27-Restaurant Guide To Eating Out.

1 tomato, sliced (5.8 g)

3 whole egg

18
Low Carb & No Carb Cookbook. (A) 130-Recipes. (B) 85-Low Carb Desserts. (C) 27-Restaurant Guide To Eating Out.

s 1/8 cup cream (1.2 g) 1/8 cup water

19
Low Carb & No Carb Cookbook. (A) 130-Recipes. (B) 85-Low Carb Desserts. (C) 27-Restaurant Guide To Eating Out.

salt & pepper to taste

4 slices bacon

Preheat oven to 450 degrees. Spray casserole dish with cooking oil. Layer tomato slices over the bottom. Beat eggs with cream & water. Beat until foamy. Stir in salt & pepper. Pour over tomatoes. Put in oven for 15 - 20 minutes. While eggs bake, cook bacon. Spray skillet with cooking spray. Cook on medium high heat. When bacon is crisp, break up bacon. Remove egg from oven (spoon off any excess tomato juice). Sprinkle bacon on top & serve.

20
Low Carb & No Carb Cookbook. (A) 130-Recipes. (B) 85-Low Carb Desserts. (C) 27-Restaurant Guide To Eating Out.

Carb Count: Recipe Total 7 g, Per Serving 3.5 g

(13) <u>HAM & CHEESE OMELET- 2 Servings</u>

6 whole eggs
2 tbs p light cream (0.5 g)
Diced lean ham
1 cup shredded cheese

Beat eggs with cream. Spray skillet with cooking spray. Cook on medium high heat. Add ham & cheese. Optional: add sliced red & green bell pepper (7.2 g per 1 cup) or other favorite omelet toppings.

Carb Count: Recipe Total 0.5 g, Per Serving 0.2 g

(14) <u>SCRAMBLED EGG PIZZA - 5 Servings</u>

1/2 cup chopped zucchini (1.9 g)

21
Low Carb & No Carb Cookbook. (A) 130-Recipes. (B) 85-Low Carb Desserts. (C) 27-Restaurant Guide To Eating Out.

1/2 cup chopped mushrooms (1.5 g)
1/8 tsp crushed red pepper
10 eggs
1/4 cup cream (2.4 g)
1/8 cup water

22
Low Carb & No Carb Cookbook. (A) 130-Recipes. (B) 85-Low Carb Desserts. (C) 27-Restaurant Guide To Eating Out.

r

1/4 cup shredded cheese
bacon, cooked, drained, crumbled

Preheat oven to 375 degrees. Sauté vegetables with red pepper for about 5 minutes, or until tender. Remove vegetables. In a large bowl, beat the eggs, cream & water together. Spray large skillet again. Add egg mixture & cook without stirring until mixture begins to set on the bottom & around the edge.
Cook a few minutes more until eggs are cooked, but still moist. Place scrambled eggs on pizza pan (sprayed with oil). Top with vegetables, bacon & cheese. Bake for 6-8 minutes, or until cheese melts.

Carb Count: Recipe Total 5.8 g, Per Serving 1.2 g

(15) SAUSAGE OR BACON BREAKFAST BURRITO - 2 Servings

Sausage or bacon
4 whole eggs
1/8 cup light

23

Low Carb & No Carb Cookbook. (A) 130-Recipes. (B) 85-Low Carb Desserts. (C) 27-Restaurant Guide To Eating Out.

cream (0.5 g) shredded cheese 1/4 cup

24
Low Carb & No Carb Cookbook. (A) 130-Recipes. (B) 85-Low Carb Desserts. (C) 27-Restaurant Guide To Eating Out.

sour cream (4 g)

2 tbsp salsa (3 g)

Cook sausage or bacon. Mix eggs with cream. Pour half of egg mixture into skillet & tip to side to spread eggs across pan. Cook thoroughly & turn egg carefully over. Repeat with remaining eggs. Divide sausage into egg "tortillas" and roll up. Top with cheese, sour cream & salsa.

Carb Count: Recipe Total 7.5 g, Per Serving 3.7 g

(16) <u>FAJITA BREAKFAST BURRITO - 2 Servings</u>

2 tsp each vinegar & soy sauce
Cubed

25
Low Carb & No Carb Cookbook. (A) 130-Recipes. (B) 85-Low Carb Desserts. (C) 27-Restaurant Guide To Eating Out.

cooked chicken
1/8 cup onion, diced (1.7 g)
1/4 cup green pepper, cut into strips (1.8 g)
Dash of cumin & garlic powder
4 eggs
1/8 cup light cream (0.5 g)
1/4 cup chedded dar

26
Low Carb & No Carb Cookbook. (A) 130-Recipes. (B) 85-Low Carb Desserts. (C) 27-Restaurant Guide To Eating Out.

cheese
1/4 cup sour cream (4 g)
2 tbsp salsa (3 g; check your brand)

In skillet, heat vinegar & soy sauce. Add chicken, onions & green peppers. Season to taste. Let cook for 3-4 minutes. Combine eggs & cream. In another skillet, cook half of egg mixture. Tilt pan to distribute evenly across pan. Let one side set & carefully turn over. Repeat with remaining egg mixture. Divide ingredients between both egg "tortillas". Top with sour cream & salsa.

Carb Count: Recipe Total 11 g, Per Serving 5 g

(17) PEACHES & RICOTTA - 4 Servings
Low Fat

2 ripe peaches, quartered, pits removed (8 g)
1/3 cup whole milk ricotta cheese (0.6 g)
1/2 cup cottage cheese (3 g)
2 packets artificial sweetener

Mix ricotta, cottage cheese & sweetener. Spoon mixture into middle of each peach. Preheat broiler. Cook under a broiler for 5-9 minutes or until peaches are hot.

Carb Count: Recipe Total 11.6 g, Per Serving 2.9 g

27
Low Carb & No Carb Cookbook. (A) 130-Recipes. (B) 85-Low Carb Desserts. (C) 27-Restaurant Guide To Eating Out.

(18) <u>**PUFFED OVEN PANCAKE - 6 Servings**</u>

2 tbsp butter

3 eggs

1/2 cup high gluten flour (12 g)
1/4 cup crea

28
Low Carb & No Carb Cookbook. (A) 130-Recipes. (B) 85-Low Carb Desserts. (C) 27-Restaurant Guide To Eating Out.

m (2.4 g) 1/4 cup water salt

Melt butter in skillet. Beat eggs. Add flour, cream, water & 1/4 tsp salt. Mix well. Pour into hot skillet. Bake at 400 degrees F for 25 minutes until puffed & golden brown. Serve with blackberry syrup, maple butter or low carb maple syrup (Recipes #25, #26, and #27).

29
Low Carb & No Carb Cookbook. (A) 130-Recipes. (B) 85-Low Carb Desserts. (C) 27-Restaurant Guide To Eating Out.

Carb Count: Recipe Total 14.2 g, Per Serving 2.5 g

(19) <u>CREPES - 6 Servings</u>

2 eggs
3/4 cup cream (7.2 g)
3/4 cup water
1 cup high gluten flour (24 g)
1 tbsp oil

Combine all ingredients. Mix well. Heat greased skillet. Pour in 2 tablespoons of batter into skillet. Tilt skillet to spread batter. Cook one side, turn. Carefully remove & repeat with remaining batter.

Carb Count: Recipe Total 31.2 g, Per Serving 5 g

(20) <u>EGGS BENEDICT - 4 Servings</u>

4 eggs
Canadian Bacon

Lightly grease skillet. Add water to half-fill skillet. Bring water to boiling. Reduce heat & simmer. Break eggs into cup & carefully slide one at a time into water. Allow each egg space. Simmer for 5 minutes. Meanwhile, heat Canadian bacon in skillet. Remove poached egg & serve with Hollandaise Sauce. For sauce, combine 1/2 cup butter, 3 beaten egg yolks, 1 tbsp water, 1 tbsp lemon

Low Carb & No Carb Cookbook. (A) 130-Recipes. (B) 85-Low Carb Desserts. (C) 27-Restaurant Guide To Eating Out.

juice (1.3 g carbs) and heat in double boiler, stirring constantly.

Carb Count: Recipe Total 1.3 g, Per Serving 0.3 g

(21) DENVER SCRAMBLED EGGS - 3 Servings

6 eggs
1/3 cup light cream (1.5 g)
1/3 cup ham, chopped

31
Low Carb & No Carb Cookbook. (A) 130-Recipes. (B) 85-Low Carb Desserts. (C) 27-Restaurant Guide To Eating Out.

3 tbsp green sweet pepper (1.5 g)
5 mushrooms, sliced (2.2 g)
shredded cheese
salt & pepper

Beat eggs with cream. Salt & pepper to taste. Melt butter in skillet. Add eggs. Cook without stirring until eggs begin to set. Add ham, vegetables & cheese. Stir mixture. Heat & serve.

Carb Count: Recipe Total 5.2 g, Per Serving 1.7 g

(22) **PUFFY OMELET WITH CHEESE SAUCE- 2 Servings**

4 eggs, se

32
Low Carb & No Carb Cookbook. (A) 130-Recipes. (B) 85-Low Carb Desserts. (C) 27-Restaurant Guide To Eating Out.

parated

2 tbsp water

salt & pepper
1 tbsp butter
1/3 cup cream

33
Low Carb & No Carb Cookbook. (A) 130-Recipes. (B) 85-Low Carb Desserts. (C) 27-Restaurant Guide To Eating Out.

(3.2g) 1/3 cup water

1/3 cup shredded cheese

Beat egg whites until frothy. Add water & continue beating until stiff. Fold egg yolks & salt & pepper into egg whites. Heat butter in an ovenproof skillet. Pour in egg mix. Cook over low heat for 10 minutes or until puffed & set on bottom. Bake at 325 degrees F for 10 minutes. While baking, combine butter, cream, water & shredded cheese in saucepan. Stir & heat until smooth. Serve omelet with cheese sauce (for a no carb meal, simply fill omelet with meat & cheese).

34
Low Carb & No Carb Cookbook. (A) 130-Recipes. (B) 85-Low Carb Desserts. (C) 27-Restaurant Guide To Eating Out.

Carb Count: Recipe Total 3.2 g, Per Serving 1.6 g

(23) <u>OVEN OMELET - 3 Servings</u>

6 eggs

1/8 cup water

salt & p

35
Low Carb & No Carb Cookbook. (A) 130-Recipes. (B) 85-Low Carb Desserts. (C) 27-Restaurant Guide To Eating Out.

epper

1/2 cup shredded cheese

3 slices bacon, cooked & crumbled

Combine eggs, water, salt & pepper. Beat well. Pour egg mixture in lightly greased pan. Bake at 400 degrees F for 5 minutes. Add cheese & bacon and bake for 5 more minutes.

36
Low Carb & No Carb Cookbook. (A) 130-Recipes. (B) 85-Low Carb Desserts. (C) 27-Restaurant Guide To Eating Out.

Carb Count: Recipe Total 0 g, Per Serving 0 g

(24) APRICOT SOUFFLES - 4 Servings *Low Fat*

3 eggs, separated
1/2 tsp lemon zest (0.1 g)
1/8 cup apricot all fruit jam (18 g)

Preheat oven to 350 degrees F. Grease four individual souffle cups. Combine egg yolks with lemon zest and apricot jam & mix well. In a separate bowl, beat egg whites until soft peaks form. Fold egg whites into yolk mixture. Pour into prepared cups & bake for 10-15 minutes.
Dust with cinnamon & serve.

Carb Count: Recipe Total 18.1 g, Per Serving 4.5 g

(25) APPLE SAUSAGE PATTIES - 4 Servings

1 egg white
1/2 cup chopped apple (10 g)
1 tbsp fresh parsley

37
Low Carb & No Carb Cookbook. (A) 130-Recipes. (B) 85-Low Carb Desserts. (C) 27-Restaurant Guide To Eating Out.

1/2 tsp salt (0.3 g)
1/4 tsp nutmeg (0.3 g)
1/4 tsp cinnamon (0.4 g)
1/2 pound sausage

Combine egg white, apple, parsley, salt, nutmeg, cinnamon, and sausage. Mix well. Shape into 8 patties. Lightly grease skillet. Cook patties for 10 minutes or until thoroughly cooked (be sure meat is not pink & juices run clear).

Carb Count: Recipe Total 11 g, Per Serving 2.7 g

(26) SPINACH PUFFS - 4 Servings *Low Fat*

2 cups spinach (4.8 g)
1/2 cup cottage cheese (3 g)
1 tsp nutm

38

Low Carb & No Carb Cookbook. (A) 130-Recipes. (B) 85-Low Carb Desserts. (C) 27-Restaurant Guide To Eating Out.

egg (1.1g) 2 egg whites 1/4 cup Parme

39
Low Carb & No Carb Cookbook. (A) 130-Recipes. (B) 85-Low Carb Desserts. (C) 27-Restaurant Guide To Eating Out.

san cheese salt & pepper

Preheat oven to 425 degrees F. Brush individual souffle dishes with oil.
Chop & cook spinach. Mix spinach with cottage cheese & add nutmeg.
Beat egg whites in a separate bowl until stiff (holding soft peaks).
Fold them into the spinach mixture and spoon into the souffle dishes. Sprinkle with Parmesan & bake for 15-20 minutes or until puffed & golden brown.

40
Low Carb & No Carb Cookbook. (A) 130-Recipes. (B) 85-Low Carb Desserts. (C) 27-Restaurant Guide To Eating Out.

Carb Count: Recipe Total 6.2 g, Per Serving 1.5 g

(27) <u>CREAMY RASPBERRY JELLO - 2 servings *Low Fat*</u>

One 3-oz package sugar free raspberry gelatin
2 c whipped cream (9 g)

Prepare gelatin according to package directions. Chill 4-6 hours before serving. Remove gelatin and beat thoroughly. Blend in whipped cream.
Chill & serve.

Carb Count: Recipe Total 9 g, Per Serving 4.5 g

(28) <u>BLUEBERRY SYRUP - 4 Servings</u>

1/2 cup frozen blackberries (9.2 g) or blueberries (10 g)
4 tbsp butter

Combine blackberries with butter in a small saucepan over low heat. Serve warm.

Carb Count: Recipe Total 9.2 g, Per Serving 2.3 g

(29)
<u>MAPLE BUTTER - 4</u>

41
Low Carb & No Carb Cookbook. (A) 130-Recipes. (B) 85-Low Carb Desserts. (C) 27-Restaurant Guide To Eating Out.

<u>Servings</u>

1 stick softened butter
4 packets artificial sweetener
1 tbsp maple extract

Mix ingredients and chill.

Carb Count: Recipe Total 0 g, Per Serving 0 g

(30) <u>MAPLE SYRUP - 4 Servings</u>

1/2 cup water
1/2 cup butter
1 package plain jello
1/2 tsp vanilla extract
1 tsp maple extract
6 packets artificial sweetener.

Bring water and butter to a boil. Add gelatin and stir until dissolved.
Remove from heat. Add extracts and sweetener.

Carb Count: Recipe Total 0 g, Per Serving 0 g

42
Low Carb & No Carb Cookbook. (A) 130-Recipes. (B) 85-Low Carb Desserts. (C) 27-Restaurant Guide To Eating Out.

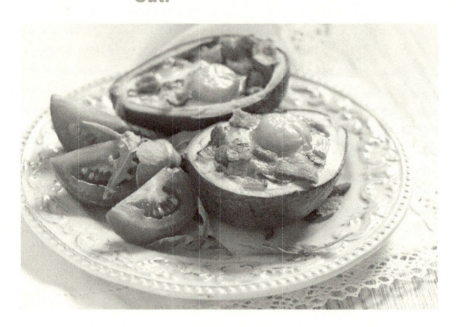

LUNCH

(31) CHEF SALAD - 2 Servings *Low Fat*

4 slices deli ham, divided
4 slices deli turkey, divided
4 slices deli roast beef, divided
1 cup

43
Low Carb & No Carb Cookbook. (A) 130-Recipes. (B) 85-Low Carb Desserts. (C) 27-Restaurant Guide To Eating Out.

cheese, divided
6 slices cucumbers (1.8 g)
Iceberg lettuce (1.6 g per cup)

Arrange meat, cheese & toppings on salad. Serve with your favorite low carb dressing. Check the label of the deli meat - sometimes sugar is added.

Carb Count: Recipe Total 3.4 g, Per Serving 1.7 g

(32) BLACKENED CHICKEN SALAD - 2 Servings *Low Fat*

Cooked, cubed chicken
2 tbsp each soy sauce & vinegar
6 slices cucumber (1.8 g)
1/4 cup chopped tomato (2.8 g)
bacon,

44
Low Carb & No Carb Cookbook. (A) 130-Recipes. (B) 85-Low Carb Desserts. (C) 27-Restaurant Guide To Eating Out.

cooked, cooled & crumbled
4 tbsp balsamic vinegar mixed with 6 tbsp olive oil, divided

Romaine lettuce (1.9 g per cup)

Combine soy sauce & vinegar. Pour into skillet. Add chicken. Heat on high until chicken chars a bit. Serve with salad. Drizzle vinegar & oil over salad.

Carb Count: Recipe Total 5.5 g, Per Serving 2.7 g

(33) <u>COBB SALAD - 2 Servings</u>

Cooked & crumbled bacon
12 boiled eggs, chopped, divided
1 cup cheese, divided
Romaine lettuce (1.9 g per cup)

45
Low Carb & No Carb Cookbook. (A) 130-Recipes. (B) 85-Low Carb Desserts. (C) 27-Restaurant Guide To Eating Out.

Arrange bacon, cheese & eggs on bed of lettuce. Enjoy with your favorite low carb dressing.

Carb Count: Recipe Total 1.9 g, Per Serving 0.8 g

(34) <u>TURKEY & CRANBERRY SALAD- 2 Servings *Low Fat*</u>

Sliced Turkey deli meat (or chicken)
Boston or Bibb lettuce (1.4 per cup)4 tbsp red wine vinegar mixed with 4 tbsp olive oil, divided (3.6 g) 1 tbsp cranberry relish (2 g)
1/4 cup chopped walnuts, divided (5 g)

Arrange turkey on bed of lettuce. Combine vinegar, oil & relish.
Drizzle vinegar & oil over salad. Sprinkle with walnuts.
Carb Count: Recipe Total 8. 4 g, Per Serving 4.2 g

(35) <u>CHICKEN NAAN - 4 Servings *Low Fat*</u>

1/8 cup p

46
Low Carb & No Carb Cookbook. (A) 130-Recipes. (B) 85-Low Carb Desserts. (C) 27-Restaurant Guide To Eating Out.

lain yogurt (1.4g) 1/2 tsp chili powde

47

Low Carb & No Carb Cookbook. (A) 130-Recipes. (B) 85-Low Carb Desserts. (C) 27-Restaurant Guide To Eating Out.

r (0.7 g) salt to taste

1 tbsp lemon juice (1.3 g)
4 portions of chicken, cooked & cubed 1/4 cup chopped tomato (2.8 g)
Romaine lettuce (1.9 g per cup)

Combine yogurt, chili powder, salt, lemon juice & cilantro. Warm chicken.
Serve with yogurt dressing, tomatoes & lettuce.

48
Low Carb & No Carb Cookbook. (A) 130-Recipes. (B) 85-Low Carb Desserts. (C) 27-Restaurant Guide To Eating Out.

Carb Count: Recipe Total 8.1 g, Per Serving 2 g

(36) <u>CHINESE CHICKEN SALAD - 4 Servings *Low Fat*</u>

3/4 tsp crushed red pepper (0.7 g)
1 garlic clove, crushed (0.9 g)
3 tbsp soy sauce
1/4 cup sesame oil
1/2 pound bean sprouts (1.5 g)
2 tbsp white vinegar
2 packets artificial sweetener
1/2 tsp dry mustard (0.1 g)
1/4 cup napa cabbage, thinly sliced (1.2 g)
1 cup romaine lettuce (1.9 g)
1 pound chicken, cooked, cut into bite sized pieces

Mix red pepper, garlic, soy sauce, sesame oil, vinegar, sweetener, and mustard. Mix lettuce & cabbage. Add chicken & dressing to lettuce beds.

Carb Count: Recipe Total 5.6 g, Per Serving 1.4 g

49
Low Carb & No Carb Cookbook. (A) 130-Recipes. (B) 85-Low Carb Desserts. (C) 27-Restaurant Guide To Eating Out.

(37) <u>BLT Salad - 2 Servings</u>

6 strips bacon, cooked
1 cup iceberg lettuce (1.6 g)
1/2 cup tomato (5.8 g)
1 tbsp mayo, divided

Place 3 strips of bacon onto lettuce with tomato & mayo.

Carb Count: Recipe Total 7.4 g, Per Serving 3.7 g

(38) <u>TURKEY & CREAM CHEESE - 2 Servings</u>

8 tbsp cream cheese, divided 2 thick slices tomato (4 g)

50 Low Carb & No Carb Cookbook. (A) 130-Recipes. (B) 85-Low Carb Desserts. (C) 27-Restaurant Guide To Eating Out.

Turkey lunch meat, divided
Spread cream cheese on tomato slice, pile on meat & enjoy. For variety, replace tomato with apple slice (1/4 apple: 5 g).

Carb Count: Recipe Total 4 g, Per Serving 2 g

(39) ITALIAN MEAT & CHEESE - 2 Servings

Salami slices
Ham slices
Provolone cheese slices
2 slices tomato (3 g)
4 tbsp balsamic vinegar mixed with 1 tbsp olive oil, divided (3.6 g)
Romaine lettuce (1.9 per cup)

Arrange meat, cheese, and tomato on lettuce. Drizzle with vinegar/oil.

Carb Count: Recipe Total 8.5 g, Per Serving 4.2 g

(40) FETA SPINACH SALAD - 4 Servings *Low Fat*

1 medium red pepper, cut into strips (8 g)
1

t
s
p

s

51
Low Carb & No Carb Cookbook. (A) 130-Recipes. (B) 85-Low Carb Desserts. (C) 27-Restaurant Guide To Eating Out.

alt 3 tbsp white vinegar black peppe

52
Low Carb & No Carb Cookbook. (A) 130-Recipes. (B) 85-Low Carb Desserts. (C) 27-Restaurant Guide To Eating Out.

r

1 cup fresh spinach (2.4 g)
8 ounces feta cheese, crumbled

Heat olive oil over medium high heat. Add red peppers & cook until tender. Remove. Add vinegar, pepper, 1 tbsp oil and 1/2 tsp salt. Add spinach & vinegar mix to bowl. Sprinkle feta cheese over all. Optional, add grill chicken.

Carb Count: Recipe Total 10.4 g, Per Serving 2.6 g

(41) ROAST BEEF & CHEESE - 2 Servings

Roast beef
S
l
i
c
e
s

c
h
e
d
d
a
r

c
h
e
e

53
Low Carb & No Carb Cookbook. (A) 130-Recipes. (B) 85-Low Carb Desserts. (C) 27-Restaurant Guide To Eating Out.

see 1/4 cup onions (3.4 g)

1/2 cup green pepper (3.6 g)

Sauté onions & green peppers. Arrange meat, cheese, onions & peppers on half a hoagie. Broil in toaster oven until cheese has melted. Serve with Horseradish Sauce (Beat 1/4 cup light cream until soft peaks form & fold in 1-2 tbsp horseradish). Optional: serve on slice of wheat bread for an additional 11 g of carbs.

54

Low Carb & No Carb Cookbook. (A) 130-Recipes. (B) 85-Low Carb Desserts. (C) 27-Restaurant Guide To Eating Out.

Carb Count: Recipe Total 7 g, Per Serving 3.5 g

(42) SPINACH WITH CHICKEN & APRICOTS - 4 Servings *Low Fat*

2 tbsp olive oil
1 tbsp balsamic vinegar (0.9 g) 1/2 tsp Dijon mustard (0.5 g)
2 apricots, pitted & sliced (8 g)
2 cups spinach (4.8 g)
1 cup feta cheese
1 pound boneless chicken, grilled
Mix oil, vinegar, mustard, 1/4 tsp salt, 1/4 tsp pepper. Stir in apricots. Toss spinach with nectarine mixture. Top with feta & chicken.

Carb Count: Recipe Total 14.2 g, Per Serving 3.7 g

(43) BUFFALO CHICKEN WINGS - 2 Servings

1 pound chi

55
Low Carb & No Carb Cookbook. (A) 130-Recipes. (B) 85-Low Carb Desserts. (C) 27-Restaurant Guide To Eating Out.

chicken wings

2 tbsp butter

1/4 cup hot pepper sauce

Bake wings at 375 degrees F for 20 minutes. In saucepan, melt butter. Stir in hot pepper sauce. Brush wings with sauce. Bake for 10 more minutes. Turnover and baste with sauce. Bake 10 more minutes. Serve with blue cheese dressing and celery (1 cup = 3.9 g).

Carb Count: Recipe Total 0 g, Per Serving 0 g

56
Low Carb & No Carb Cookbook. (A) 130-Recipes. (B) 85-Low Carb Desserts. (C) 27-Restaurant Guide To Eating Out.

(44) TUNA MELT - 2 Servings *Low Fat*

2 cans water-packed tuna, drained
1/2 cup cottage cheese (3 g)
4 tbsp mayo
3 tsp lemon juice (0.9 g) dash garlic powder Cheese slices
Celery (1 cup = 3.9 g)

Combine tuna with cottage cheese, mayo, lemon juice & garlic powder.
Heat on skillet.
Enjoy with cheese and celery.

Carb Count: Recipe Total 7.8 g, Per Serving 3.9 g

57
Low Carb & No Carb Cookbook. (A) 130-Recipes. (B) 85-Low Carb Desserts. (C) 27-Restaurant Guide To Eating Out.

(45) CHICKEN & PROVOLONE SALAD - 5 Servings *Low Fat*

1 tbsp chopped fresh basil (1.5 g)
1 1/2 tbsp olive oil
1 tbsp lemon juice (1.3 g)
1 tsp

58
Low Carb & No Carb Cookbook. (A) 130-Recipes. (B) 85-Low Carb Desserts. (C) 27-Restaurant Guide To Eating Out.

Dijon Mustard (1 g)

1/2 tsp oregano (0.5 g)
1/2 pound grilled chicken, cut up
1/4 cup diced tomato (2.9 g)
1/2 pound fresh provolone, sliced

Mix basil, olive oil, lemon juice, dijon mustard & oregano. Layer chicken, tomato & cheese. Drizzle dressing over all.

59
Low Carb & No Carb Cookbook. (A) 130-Recipes. (B) 85-Low Carb Desserts. (C) 27-Restaurant Guide To Eating Out.

Carb Count: Recipe Total 7.2 g, Per Serving 1.4 g

(46) SMOKED SALMON MUFFINS - 6 Servings

1 cup high gluten flour (24 g)
1 tsp baking powder
1 cup cream (9.6 g)
1/2 cup water
6 eggs beaten
1 cup cheese, shredded
1/2 cup smoked salmon

Preheat oven to 400 degrees. Combine flour & baking powder. In a separate bowl, combine milk, egg & cheese. Mix wet & dry ingredients. Stir in salmon. Pour into muffin tin. Bake for 10-15 minutes.

Carb Count: Recipe Total 33.6 g, Per Serving 5.5 g

(47) BEEF MINESTRONE - 6 Servings
Low Fat

16 ounces can of chopped tomatoes, undrained (21 g)
1 large carrot, grated (7 g)
1/2 cup chopped cauliflower (2.2 g)
2 cubes beef bouillon
1/2 pound extra lean ground beef or turkey
minced garlic to taste (1 clove 0.9 g)

In large pot, combine tomatoes, carrots, bouillon & pasta. Bring to a boil & reduce

60

Low Carb & No Carb Cookbook. (A) 130-Recipes. (B) 85-Low Carb Desserts. (C) 27-Restaurant Guide To Eating Out.

heat & simmer. In separate skillet, cook meat with garlic.
Drain fat from meat (pat with paper towels).
Transfer meat to pot.
Heat & serve.

Carb Count: Recipe Total 31 g, Per Serving 5.1 g

(48) BEEF JERKY - 4 Servings *Low Fat*

1 lb. beef, sliced
1/2 cup soy sauce
3 tbsp. liquid smoke
1/8

61
Low Carb & No Carb Cookbook. (A) 130-Recipes. (B) 85-Low Carb Desserts. (C) 27-Restaurant Guide To Eating Out.

cup water

1 clove fresh garlic (0.9 g) 1 tspoon onion powder (1.6

62
Low Carb & No Carb Cookbook. (A) 130-Recipes. (B) 85-Low Carb Desserts. (C) 27-Restaurant Guide To Eating Out.

g) sugar substitute equal to 2 tsp

Slice beef into slices. Absorb any excess water with paper towels. Combine all ingredients (except beef). Marinate for several hours (can do overnight). When you're ready, to make the jerky, place the beef onto a cookie sheet sprayed with cooking spray (or a dehydrator tray - if using, follow drying instructions). Preheat oven to 200 degrees F. Cook for several hours until dry, but still chewy (not crunchy). Turn the strips once every hour until done. For pepper jerky, add 1 tbsp fresh pepper (5.2 g). For chili jerky, add 1 tbsp chili powder (4.4 g).

Carb Count: Recipe Total 2.5 g, Per Serving 0.6 g

63
Low Carb & No Carb Cookbook. (A) 130-Recipes. (B) 85-Low Carb Desserts. (C) 27-Restaurant Guide To Eating Out.

(49) WALDORF CHICKEN SALAD- 3 Servings

2 cans chicken, drained
1 package cream cheese
1/2 apple chopp

64
Low Carb & No Carb Cookbook. (A) 130-Recipes. (B) 85-Low Carb Desserts. (C) 27-Restaurant Guide To Eating Out.

e
d
(
1
0
g
)
1 celery stalk, chopped (1.5 g)

Combine all ingredients & enjoy.

Carb Count: Recipe Total 11.5 g, Per Serving 3.8 g

(50) <u>SEAFOOD SALAD- 2 Servings *Low</u>

Fat* 2 tbsp sliced green onions (0.3 g) minced garlic to taste (0.9 g per clove)
1 cup sliced mushroom (3.1 g)
1/2 pound shrimp, cooked
Sauté onion & garlic. Add mushrooms & shrimp. Serve with mayonnaise & toasted pita triangles (5 g for half a pita pocket).

Carb Count: Recipe Total 4.3 g, Per Serving 2.1 g

(51) <u>SALMON PATTIE</u>

65

Low Carb & No Carb Cookbook. (A) 130-Recipes. (B) 85-Low Carb Desserts. (C) 27-Restaurant Guide To Eating Out.

S- 4 Serving

16 ounce can Salmon
pinch of salt
1/2 cup green onion, diced (3.7 g)
4 tbsp pork rinds, crushed
8 eggs
1 tsp lemon juice (0.3 g)

Preheat oven to 400 degrees. Mix all the ingredients together in a bowl. Form into patties about 1/2 to 3/4-inch-thick and 2 1/2 - 3 inches diameter. This should make about 8 patties. Bake in a pan sprayed with cooking oil until brown (about 15 minutes). Can be served hot or cold (great for a lunch on the go). Serve with your favorite carbs (asparagus is a nice side for a hot sit-down meal; cauliflower & cheese slices are nice in a lunch box).

Carb Count: Recipe Total 4 g, Per Serving 1 g

(52) ZUCCHINI BOATS - 4 Servings *Low Fat*

4 zucchinis (10 g)
1/4 cup chopped green onion (1.8 g)
1/2 green bell pepper, chopped (3.6 g)
4 whole eggs
2 tbsp cream (1.2 g)

Low Carb & No Carb Cookbook. (A) 130-Recipes. (B) 85-Low Carb Desserts. (C) 27-Restaurant Guide To Eating Out.

1/2 cup shredded cheese

Preheat oven to 375 degrees. Slice zucchini in half & scoop out middle, leaving 8 "boats". Steam boats for 5 minutes. Meanwhile, chop up leftover zucchini and sauté in a large skillet with onion & bell pepper until soft. Combine zucchini/onion/bell pepper mixture with eggs & cream. Place zucchini/egg mix in boats. Sprinkle with cheese. Bake in oven until heated throughout & cheese is melted.

Carb Count: Recipe Total 16.6 g, Per Serving 4.1 g

(53) STUFFED MUSHROOMS - 3 Servings *Low Fat*

12 large fresh mushrooms (6 g)
2 tbsp sliced green onions (0.3 g)
1/2 clove garlic, crushed (0.4 g)
1/8 cup butter
1/2 cup shr

67
Low Carb & No Carb Cookbook. (A) 130-Recipes. (B) 85-Low Carb Desserts. (C) 27-Restaurant Guide To Eating Out.

edded cheese 1/4 cup ham

1 tbsp cream cheese

Rinse & drain mushrooms. Remove stems and chop up. Combine stems, onions, garlic, & butter. Heat in saucepan. Stir in cheese, ham & cream cheese. Spoon into mushroom caps. Bake at 400 degrees F for 10 minutes.

Carb Count: Recipe Total 6.7 g, Per Serving 2.2 g

(54) SALMON AND CUCUMBER - 3 Servings

68
Low Carb & No Carb Cookbook. (A) 130-Recipes. (B) 85-Low Carb Desserts. (C) 27-Restaurant Guide To Eating Out.

4 ounces smoked salmon, flaked
4 ounces cream cheese
1 tbsp sliced green onion (0.1 g)
2 tsp fresh dill (1 g)
1 tbsp lemon juice (1.3 g)
1 cucumber, cut into 12 slices (3.6 g)

Mix all ingredients except for cucumber. Spread salmon on cucumber.

Carb Count: Recipe Total 6 g, Per Serving 2 g

(55) TUNA SPREAD - 2 Servings

1/2 cup cr

69
Low Carb & No Carb Cookbook. (A) 130-Recipes. (B) 85-Low Carb Desserts. (C) 27-Restaurant Guide To Eating Out.

eam cheese

3 tbsp mayonnaise

1 clove garlic, minced (0.9 g)
1/8 tsp red pepper (0.1 g)
6.5 ounce can tuna, drained, broken up
1/8 cup chopped red pepper (2 g)

Mix all ingredients. Serve with celery (1 cup = 3.9 g) and cheese.

70
Low Carb & No Carb Cookbook. (A) 130-Recipes. (B) 85-Low Carb Desserts. (C) 27-Restaurant Guide To Eating Out.

Carb Count: Recipe Total 3 g, Per Serving 1.5 g

(56) CHILI CHEESE BURGERS - 2 Servings

1 pound hamburger
1 egg
1/2 tbsp chili powder (2.4 g)
1/2 cup shredded cheese

Combine all ingredients. Grill and serve with lettuce (1.6 g per cup), sour cream (16 g per cup) and salsa (1.5 g per tablespoon).

Carb Count: Recipe Total 2.4 g, Per Serving 1.2 g

(57) GOAT CHEESE WITH SPINACH & SUNDRIED TOMATOES - 4 Servings

1 cup romaine lettuce (1.9 g)
1/2 cup spinach (1.2 g)
1 radish, diced (0.2 g)
4 tbsp sundried tomatoes (1.5 g)
3 tbsp olive oil
1 tbsp balsamic vinegar (0.9 g)
1/2 pound goat cheese

71
Low Carb & No Carb Cookbook. (A) 130-Recipes. (B) 85-Low Carb Desserts. (C) 27-Restaurant Guide To Eating Out.

Slice goat cheese with oil & broil until golden. Serve on top of salad with radish, tomatoes & oil and vinegar drizzled over all.

Carb Count: Recipe Total 4.7 g, Per Serving 1.1 g

(58) <u>SOUTHWEST HAMBURGER - 2 Servings</u>

1 pounds hamburger
1 garlic clove,
   minced (0.9 g)
1/2 tbsp each chili powder (2.4 g) and vinegar
2 tsp cumin (1.8 g)
   salt and pepper to
   taste

Combine all ingredients. Grill and serve with lettuce (1.6 g per cup), sour cream (16 g per cup) and salsa (1.5 g per tablespoon).

Carb Count: Recipe Total 3.1 g, Per Serving 1.5 g

(59) <u>CHILI CHEESE HOT DOGS - 2 Servings</u>

No Carb Hot Dogs (check label)
1/4 cup onions, chopped (3.4 g)
1/2 cup cheese
1 cup Low Carb Chili (Dinner Recipe #67) (2.5 g)

Sauté onions in oil. Heat chili. Cook hot dogs according to package

72
Low Carb & No Carb Cookbook. (A) 130-Recipes. (B) 85-Low Carb Desserts. (C) 27-Restaurant Guide To Eating Out.

directions. Serve with chili, cheese & sautéed onions.

Carb Count: Recipe Total 5.9 g, Per Serving 2.9 g

(60) <u>HAMBURGER PIZZA - 2 Servings</u>

1/2 pound hamburger

1 egg

2 tsp pizza spice blend (1 g)
1/8 cup pizza sauce (2 g;

73
Low Carb & No Carb Cookbook. (A) 130-Recipes. (B) 85-Low Carb Desserts. (C) 27-Restaurant Guide To Eating Out.

check your label)
2 tbsp olives (2 g)
1/8 cup green bell peppers, diced (0.8 g)
shredded cheese

Combine all ingredients. Grill and serve with salad.

Carb Count: Recipe Total 5.8 g, Per Serving 2.9 g

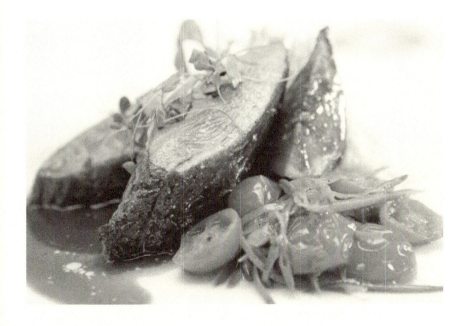

DINNER

74
Low Carb & No Carb Cookbook. (A) 130-Recipes. (B) 85-Low Carb Desserts. (C) 27-Restaurant Guide To Eating Out.

(61) GRILLED SESAME SALMON - 4 Servings

2 six-ounce salmon fillets, all skin removed salt & pepper
4 tbsp sesame seeds (5.6 g)
3 tsp olive oil
2 tbsp rice wine vinegar (1.8 g)
2 tbsp soy sauce
2 cucumbers, sliced thinly lengthwise (6 g)

Heat grill or broiler. Slice the salmon fillets open horizontally, leave one end intact. Spread fillets open and turn over. Season with salt & pepper. Tightly roll fillets. Secure with toothpick. Pour sesame seeds into a

75
Low Carb & No Carb Cookbook. (A) 130-Recipes. (B) 85-Low Carb Desserts. (C) 27-Restaurant Guide To Eating Out.

small dish. Place rolled fillets in the seeds & coat bottom. Drizzle with olive oil. In a small bowl, mix vinegar & soy sauce. Set aside. Fold edges of a piece of heavy-duty aluminum foil to form a shallow baking pan; place on grill. Arrange rolled fillets on foil. Grill 4-6 minutes on each side (or broil in the oven). Remove, drizzle with reserved soy mixture & place on bed of cucumber strips. Serve with brown rice.
Carb Count: Recipe Total 13.4 g, Per Serving 3.3 g

(62) CHICKEN PARMESAN - 4 Servings

4 Chicken Breasts
2 eggs, beaten
1 cup pork rinds, crushed 1/2 cup mushrooms (2.3 g carbs)
1/2 cup spaghetti sauce (8 g, check your brand)

Dip the chicken in the eggs and then coat with the pork rinds. Heat olive oil in pan & fry up the chicken. Sauté the mushrooms. Serve with spaghetti sauce and cheese (if desired, place in baking dish & bake at 375 degrees F for 30 minutes or until cheese is bubbly).

Carb Count: Recipe Total 10.3 g, Per Serving 2.5 g

(63) CHICKEN WITH PEANUT SAUCE - 4 Servings *Low Fat*

2 pounds boneless chicken

76
Low Carb & No Carb Cookbook. (A) 130-Recipes. (B) 85-Low Carb Desserts. (C) 27-Restaurant Guide To Eating Out.

1/4 cup peanut butter (12 g; check your brand)
2 tbsp soy sauce
1 tsp white vinegar
1/8 tsp crushed red pepper (0.1)
2/3 cup water

Heat vegetable oil over medium high heat. Add chicken and cook until golden brown. Remove. Mix remaining ingredients and add to skillet.
Stir until heated through. Serve sauce with chicken.

Carb Count Recipe Total: 12.1 g Per Serving: 3 g

(64) CHICKEN TIKKA SALAD - 4 Servings *Low Fat*

This is a quick & easy Indian salad.
3 chicken breasts
1 tsp ground ginger (1.3 g)
1/2 garlic clove, crushed (0.4 g)
1/2 tsp chili powder (0.

77

Low Carb & No Carb Cookbook. (A) 130-Recipes. (B) 85-Low Carb Desserts. (C) 27-Restaurant Guide To Eating Out.

7 g)
1/2 tsp salt
1/2 cup plain yogurt (5.3 g)
4 tbsp lemon juice (5.2 g)
1 tbsp fresh cilantro, chopped (0.3 g)
1 tbsp olive oil
1 cup romaine lettuce (1.9 g)
Lime wedges

Combine all ingredients. Marinate chicken for at least 2 hours. Reserve marinade. Preheat broiler. Broil chicken 15-20 minutes, basting 2-3 times. Serve with favorite dressing.

Carb Count: Recipe Total 16.1 g, Per Serving 4 g

(65) MARSALA CHICKEN – 4 Servings *Low Fat*

2 pounds boneless chicken salt & pepper to taste
1 cup fresh mushrooms (3.1 g)
1/4 cup Marsala wine (5 g)

Heat olive oil over medium high heat. Add chicken and cook until golden brown. Sprinkle with salt & pepper. Reduce heat to medium. Cook thoroughly. Remove. Add mushrooms to same skillet & cook until

78
Low Carb & No Carb Cookbook. (A) 130-Recipes. (B) 85-Low Carb Desserts. (C) 27-Restaurant Guide To Eating Out.

golden brown. Add wine to mushrooms. Return chicken. Heat & serve.

Carb Count: Recipe Total 8.1 g, Per Serving 2 g

(66) MUSTARD CHICKEN - 4 serving
Low Fat

1/3 cup Dijon mustard (12 g)
2 tbsp chopped fresh dill (or 1 tbsp dried dill) (4 g)
1 tsp freshly grated orange peel (0.5 g)
4 skinless, boneless chicken breasts

Preheat oven to 400 degrees. Combine mustard & honey in a small bowl. Stir in dill & orange peel. Line a baking sheet with foil. Brush sauce on top of chicken. Bake until thoroughly cooked, about 30 minutes.

Carb Count: Recipe Total 16.5 g, Per Serving 4.1 g

(67) SLOPPY JOES - 6 Servings

1 pound extra lean ground beef or turkey
1 7 1/2 oz can tomatoes, diced (9 g)
1/4 cup water
1 tsp chili powder (1.4 g)
2 tsp Worcestershire sauce
1
/
2

79
Low Carb & No Carb Cookbook. (A) 130-Recipes. (B) 85-Low Carb Desserts. (C) 27-Restaurant Guide To Eating Out.

t s p

garlic salt

dash

hot

pepper

sauc

e

In a large skillet, cook meat until brown. Drain off fat (remove from skillet and pat meat with paper towels). Return to skillet & stir in undrained tomatoes, water, chili powder, Worcestershire sauce, garlic salt & hot pepper sauce). Bring to a boil. Reduce heat, simmer, for 5-10 minutes or until desired consistency. (Optional: serve with half a hamburger bun for an additional 5 g of carbs).

Carb Count: Recipe Total 10.4 g, Per Serving 1.7 g

(68) POT ROAST - 8 Servings *Low Fat*

2 pound boneless venison shoulder or rump roast
1 tbsp cooking oil
1/2 cup soy sauce
2 1/2 cups of water

Trim fat from meat. In pot, brown meat in oil. Drain off fat. Add soy sauce & water. Bring to a boil. Reduce heat. Simmer, covered for 1 1/2 -2 hours. Serve with steamed cauliflower (1 cup = 5.1 g) with melted cheese.

Carb Count: Recipe Total 0 g, Per Serving 0 g

(69) BACON-CHICKEN ROLLS - 4 Servings

8 slices bacon, cooked & crumbled

81
Low Carb & No Carb Cookbook. (A) 130-Recipes. (B) 85-Low Carb Desserts. (C) 27-Restaurant Guide To Eating Out.

1/4 cup Parmesan cheese
2 tbsp fresh parsley (0.6 g)
1/2 tsp dried oregano (0.5 g)
1 pound boneless chicken
2 tbsp oil
salt
2 c chicken broth
1/2 cup diced tomato (5.8 g)

Mix bacon, Parmesan cheese, and herbs. Flatten chicken and fill with half of the bacon mix. Roll up and secure with a toothpick. In skillet, heat oil. Add chicken and salt and cook until golden brown. Remove. Add broth & tomatoes and heat to boiling. Add remaining bacon mix. Reduce heat and simmer on low for 5 minutes. Return chicken roll, heat and serve.

Carb Count: Recipe Total 6.9 g, Per Serving 1.8 g

(70) STUFFED GREEN PEPPERS - 4 Servings

2 large green peppers (14 g)
1 pound ground beef
7 1/2 ounce canned tomatoes, diced (9 g)
1 tbsp Worcestershire sauce
1/2 tsp

dried oregano (0.5 g)
shredded cheddar cheese

Halve peppers lengthwise, removing stem ends, seeds & membranes. Immerse in boiling water for 3 minutes Invert on paper towels & drain well. In a large skillet cook meat until brown. Drain off fat (remove & pat with paper towels). Return meat to skillet & stir in undrained tomatoes, Worcestershire sauce, oregano, salt and pepper to taste. Bring to a boil. Reduce heat & simmer for 15 minutes. Stir in half of the cheese. Fill peppers with meat mixture. Place in 2-quart baking dish. Bake at 375 degrees for 15 minutes. Sprinkle with remaining cheese. Let stand 2 minutes.

Carb Count: Recipe Total 23.5 g, Per Serving: 5.8 g

(71) MEDITERRANEAN CHICKEN - 4 Servings *Low Fat*

4 chicken breasts, cut into bite sized cubes
1 garlic clove, minced (0.9 g)
7 ounces can

83
Low Carb & No Carb Cookbook. (A) 130-Recipes. (B) 85-Low Carb Desserts. (C) 27-Restaurant Guide To Eating Out.

stewed tomatoes (9 g) 1 cup
zucchini, diced (3.8 g)
1/2 green pepper, diced (3.6 g)
2 tbsp sliced olives (1 g)
1/2 tsp dried oregano, crushed (0.5 g) salt & pepper to taste

Spray skillet with cooking spray. Cook chicken with garlic on medium heat. Add undrained tomatoes with vegetables & seasoning. Bring to a boil. Reduce heat & simmer (covered) for 30-40 minutes. Uncover & simmer for 5-10 more minutes until sauce is thickened.

Carb Count: Recipe Total 18.8, Per Serving 4.7 g

(72) APRICOT GLAZED PORK MEDALLIONS - 4 Servings *Low Fat*

1 pound pork medallions
1/4 tsp each salt & pepper
1/3 cup no sugar apricot preserves (10 g; check your brand)
2 tsp Worcestershire sauce

Stir together preserves and Worcestershire sauce. Set aside. Rub pork with salt, pepper &

Low Carb & No Carb Cookbook. (A) 130-Recipes. (B) 85-Low Carb Desserts. (C) 27-Restaurant Guide To Eating Out.

oil. Heat oil in skillet. Cook pork until no longer pink. Add apricot sauce and stir fry until a glaze forms. Serve with steamed cauliflower (1 cup cooked 5.1 g) or buttered asparagus (1/4 pound
2.2 g) or sautéed squash (1 cup cooked 6.5 g) with zucchini (1/2 cup 1.9g). Glaze is also good over roasted pork.

Carb Count: Recipe Total 10 g, Per Serving 2.5 g

(73) CHICKEN WITH OLIVES - 4 Serving
Low Fat

2 pounds boneless chicken
salt
1/2 cup chopped onion (6.9 g)
1 cup chicken broth
4 tbsp sliced olives (2 g)
1 tsp fresh thyme, chopped (1 g)

Heat olive oil in skillet. Add chicken & sprinkle with salt. Cook until light brown & remove. Add onions to skillet & cook until translucent.
Add broth, olives, thyme and chicken. Reduce heat; cover and simmer 20-25 minutes.

Carb Count: Recipe Total 9.9 g, Per Serving: 2.4 g

(74) ARTICHOKE SOUP - 3 Servings

85
Low Carb & No Carb Cookbook. (A) 130-Recipes. (B) 85-Low Carb Desserts. (C) 27-Restaurant Guide To Eating Out.

1/2 pound artichokes, peeled (14 g)
3 cup chicken broth, divided
4 tbs plight cream (1.1 g)
salt & pepper to taste

Place artichokes in a saucepan & cover with cold water. Bring to a boil. Cover & simmer until completely soft. Cool in the

86
Low Carb & No Carb Cookbook. (A) 130-Recipes. (B) 85-Low Carb Desserts. (C) 27-Restaurant Guide To Eating Out.

liquid, then drain. Place the artichokes in a blender or food processor, add half of the chicken broth & puree until smooth. Gradually add remaining stock. Stir in light cream & season to taste. Serve with protein portion (grilled fish or chicken recommended).

Carb Count: Recipe Total 15.1 g, Per Serving 5 g

(75) GREEK CHICKEN - 4 Servings *Low Fat*

1 pound boneless chicken
1 cup crumbled feta cheese
1/2 tsp dried oregano (0.5 g)
1 tbsp lemon juice (1.3 g)
1

t
b
s
p

o
i
l

s
a
l
t

&

p

87
Low Carb & No Carb Cookbook. (A) 130-Recipes. (B) 85-Low Carb Desserts. (C) 27-Restaurant Guide To Eating Out.

epper to taste

1 cup chicken broth

1/2 cup tomato diced (5.8 g)
1 cup fresh spinach (2.4 g)

88
Low Carb & No Carb Cookbook. (A) 130-Recipes. (B) 85-Low Carb Desserts. (C) 27-Restaurant Guide To Eating Out.

Flatten chicken. Combine feta, lemon juice and oregano. Spread over chicken. Fold chicken to enclose filling; secure with a toothpick. Heat oil in a skillet until hot. Add chicken and cook until golden brown.
Mix chicken broth, tomato and spinach. Add to skillet, heat to boiling.
Reduce heat to low; cover & simmer 8-10 minutes. Serve.

Carb Count: Recipe Total 10 g, Per Serving: 2.5 g

(76) <u>TURKEY WITH BACON - 4 Serving *Low Fat*</u>

4 slices bacon, cut into pieces
1 cup sliced mushrooms (3.1 g)2 pounds boneless turkey
1 cup chicken broth

Cook bacon over medium heat until browned. Remove. Cook mushrooms in bacon fat over high heat, until tender. Remove. In same pan, cook turkey until brown. Add chicken broth the turkey. Heat to boiling. Reduce heat to low; cover and simmer 20 minutes. Return mushrooms & bacon to skillet. Heat & serve.

Carb Count: Recipe Total 3.1 g, Per Serving 0.8 g

(77) <u>TERIYAKI BEEF - 4 Servings *Low Fat*</u>

89
Low Carb & No Carb Cookbook. (A) 130-Recipes. (B) 85-Low Carb Desserts. (C) 27-Restaurant Guide To Eating Out.

1 cup oil
2 tsp ginger (2.6 g)
4 packets artificial sweetener
1 cup soy sauce
1/4 cup sherry
2 cloves garlic, diced (1.8 g)
1/4 cup scallions, diced (2.5 g carbs)
1 pound beef, thinly sliced

Mix all ingredients except beef. Marinate meat in sauce for several hours. Stir fry beef. Serve with steamed, buttered asparagus (6 fresh stalks are just 2.4 g carbs) or steamed, buttered cauliflower (1 c is just 2.6 g carbs).

Carb Count: Recipe Total 6.9 g, Per Serving 1.7 g

(78) DIJON PORK WITH GRAPES - 4 Servings *Low Fat*

4 pork chops
1/2 cup light

90
Low Carb & No Carb Cookbook. (A) 130-Recipes. (B) 85-Low Carb Desserts. (C) 27-Restaurant Guide To Eating Out.

cream (2.4g)

1 tbsp Dijon mustard (

91
Low Carb & No Carb Cookbook. (A) 130-Recipes. (B) 85-Low Carb Desserts. (C) 27-Restaurant Guide To Eating Out.

4

g
)

1/2 tbsp yellow mustard (0.6 g)
1/2 cup grapes, sliced (13.5 g)

Heat olive oil over medium high heat until hot. Add pork chops and cook until golden. Transfer to a plate. Add cream, mustard and grapes. Heat until well combined. Pour sauce over pork chops and serve.

Carb Count: Recipe Total 20.5 g, Per Serving: 5.1 g

(79) BBQ CHICKEN - 4 Servings *Low Fat*

4 tbsp soy sauce
3 tbsp balsamic vinegar (2.7 g)
2

t
s
p

l
e
m
o
n

j
u

92
Low Carb & No Carb Cookbook. (A) 130-Recipes. (B) 85-Low Carb Desserts. (C) 27-Restaurant Guide To Eating Out.

ice (0.4 g)

4 tbsp tomato paste

1 clove garlic, diced (0.9 g)
1 tsp liquid

93

Low Carb & No Carb Cookbook. (A) 130-Recipes. (B) 85-Low Carb Desserts. (C) 27-Restaurant Guide To Eating Out.

smoke flavoring
1/2 cup oil
4 tsp cayenne (4.0 g)
4 chicken breasts

Combine all ingredients except chicken. Marinate chicken in sauce for at least 2 hours.
Bake for 40 minutes at 375 degrees F or grill.
Carb Count: Recipe Total 8.8 g, Per Serving 2.2 g

(80) CARIBBEAN CHICKEN KABOBS - 4 servings *Low Fat*

4 skinless, boneless chicken breasts
1 lime rind, finely grated (0.6 g)
2 tbsp lime juice (2.8 g) 1 tbsp rum
1 tsp cinnamon (1.8 g)
Cut chicken into bite sized chunks. Place in a bowl with the lime rind, juice, rum, sugar & cinnamon. Marinate 1 hour. Save the juices & thread chicken on 4 wooden skewers. Cook the skewers under a broiler or grill for 8-10 minutes, turning occasionally & basting with the juices. Serve with small salad.

94
Low Carb & No Carb Cookbook. (A) 130-Recipes. (B) 85-Low Carb Desserts. (C) 27-Restaurant Guide To Eating Out.

Carb Count: Recipe Total 5.2 g, Per Serving 1.3 g

(81) <u>TUSCAN CHICKEN CASSEROLE - 4 servings *Low Fat*</u>

4 skinless, boneless chicken breasts 1/4 cup chopped onion (3.4 g)
1 red bell pepper, seeded, sliced (8 g)
1 crushed garlic clove (0.9 g)
1 cup pureed tomatoes (10 g) 2/3 cup dry white wine
1 tsp dried

95
Low Carb & No Carb Cookbook. (A) 130-Recipes. (B) 85-Low Carb Desserts. (C) 27-Restaurant Guide To Eating Out.

d oregano (1 g) 1/2 cup crushed pork r

96
Low Carb & No Carb Cookbook. (A) 130-Recipes. (B) 85-Low Carb Desserts. (C) 27-Restaurant Guide To Eating Out.

inds

shredded

cheese

salt & pepper to taste

Spray skillet with cooking spray. Cook the chicken until golden brown. Remove. Add onions & bell peppers to the pan & sauté until softened but not brown. Stir in the garlic. Add chicken, tomatoes, wine & oregano. Bring to a boil, then cover the skillet. Lower the heat & simmer, stirring occasionally for 30-35 minutes. Sprinkle with pork rinds and cheese. Cook under broiler until golden brown (use oven safe skillet or transfer to casserole dish). Serve with small salad.

Carb Count: Recipe Total 23.3 g, Per Serving 5.8 g

97
Low Carb & No Carb Cookbook. (A) 130-Recipes. (B) 85-Low Carb Desserts. (C) 27-Restaurant Guide To Eating Out.

(82) THAI CHICKEN STIR FRY - 4 Servings
Low Fat

1/2 lemon rind, sliced (0.6 g)
2 tsp ground ginger (2.6 g)
1 garlic clove, chopped (0.9 g)
4 boneless chicken breasts, cut into bite-sized pieces
1/2 red bell pepper, seeded & sliced (4 g)
1 medium carrot, cut into match sticks (5 g)
2 tbsp oyster sauce
   salt & pepper
4 tbsp fresh cilantro (0.5 g)

Spray skillet with cooking spray. Stir fry lemon rind with garlic & ginger until brown. Add chicken & stir fry for a few minutes. Add vegetables & stir-fry until chicken is cooked & vegetables are almost cooked. Stir in oyster sauce & season to taste. Stir-fry one more minute. Garnish with cilantro.

Carb Count: Recipe Total 13.6 g, Per Serving 3.4 g

(83) ORANGE BEEF STIR FRY- 4 Servings *Low Fat*

1 pound lean beef fillet or sirloin cut into strips grated rind & juice of 1 orange (10 g for marinade; approx. 3 g as consumed)
1 tbsp soy sauce
1 tsp cornstarch
2 tsp ground ginger (2.6 g)
2 tsp sesame oil
1 medium carrot, cut into matchsticks (6 g)
1/4 cup green onions, sliced (0.8 g)

Marinate beef in orange rind & juice for 30-40 minutes. Drain liquid from the meat & set aside. Mix meat with soy sauce, cornstarch & ginger. Spray skillet with cooking spray. Stir fry beef for a few minutes. Add carrots & stir-fry a few minutes more. Stir in green onions & reserved liquid. Cook, stirring, until boiling & thickened.

Carb Count: Recipe Total 12.4 g, Per Serving 3.1 g

99
Low Carb & No Carb Cookbook. (A) 130-Recipes. (B) 85-Low Carb Desserts. (C) 27-Restaurant Guide To Eating Out.

(84) LEMON FISH - 4 Servings *Low Fat*

4 white fish fillets
1 tbsp oil
1 tbsp fresh lemon juice (1.3 g)
1 garlic clove, thinly sliced (0.9 g)
4 tbsp whole milk ricotta cheese (1 g)
4 tbsp low fat plain yogurt (2.8 g)
1 tbsp fresh chives, optional (0.6 g)

Preheat oven to 400 degrees. Place fish in aluminum foil packet with oil, garlic & lemon juice. Place fish packet in oven. Mix the ricotta cheese with yogurt & stir in snipped chives. When fish is done, remove & serve with ricotta/yogurt sauce.

Carb Count: Recipe Total 6.6 g, Per Serving 1.6 g

(85) CHICKEN STUFFED WITH SUNDRIED TOMATOES - 4 Servings *Low Fat*

1/4 cup oil-packed sundried tomatoes (2 g)
1 tsp basil (0.9 g)
1/4 cup Parmesan cheese
4 chicken breast halves

Preheat oven to 425 degrees F. Chop tomatoes & mix with basil, Parmesan (salt & pepper to

100
Low Carb & No Carb Cookbook. (A) 130-Recipes. (B) 85-Low Carb Desserts. (C) 27-Restaurant Guide To Eating Out.

taste). Cut a pocket into each chicken breast. Stuff with tomato mixture. Sprinkle with salt & pepper. Bake 35-40 minutes.

Carb Count: Recipe Total 2.9 g, Per Serving 0.7 g

(86) <u>CHICKEN STUFFED WITH BACON - 4 Servings</u>

8 slices bacon, cooked & crumbled
1/8 cup spinach (0.3 g)
1/4 cup mozzarella cheese
1/4 cup ricotta cheese (2 g)
4 chicken breast halves
Preheat oven to 425 degrees F. Combine bacon with spinach & cheeses.
Cut a pocket into each chicken breast. Stuff with bacon mixture.
Sprinkle with salt & pepper. Bake 35-40 minutes.

Carb Count: Recipe Total 2.3 g, Per Serving 0.5 g

(87) <u>CHICKEN STUFFED WITH PROSCIUTTO - 4 Servings</u>

Prosciutto, chopped
1/2 tbs p le mo n juic e

101
Low Carb & No Carb Cookbook. (A) 130-Recipes. (B) 85-Low Carb Desserts. (C) 27-Restaurant Guide To Eating Out.

(0.5 g)
1/4 cup cream cheese
4 chicken breast halves

Preheat oven to 425 degrees F. Combine prosciutto, lemon juice & cream cheese. Cut a pocket into each chicken breast. Stuff with prosciutto mixture. Sprinkle with salt & pepper. Bake 35-40 minutes.

Carb Count: Recipe Total 0.5 g, Per Serving 0.1 g

(88) STUFFED TURKEY ROLLS - 4 Servings

4 turkey breasts
4 slices Swiss cheese
4 tsp tomato paste (2.5 g)
1/4 cup fresh spinach (0.6 g)
1 crushed garlic clove

102
Low Carb & No Carb Cookbook. (A) 130-Recipes. (B) 85-Low Carb Desserts. (C) 27-Restaurant Guide To Eating Out.

(0.9 g) 1 tbsp light cream (0.3 g)
salt & pepper

Flatten turkey slightly with a rolling pin. Spread tomato paste, cheese, spinach & crushed garlic on each turkey breast. Add salt & pepper. Roll up around filling & secure with a toothpick. Place spirals on a foil-lined broiler pan. Broil for 15-20 minutes, turning every 5 minutes, until thoroughly cooked.

Carb Count: Recipe Total 4.3 g, Per Serving 1.1 g

(89) GRILLED SESAME CHICKEN - 4 Servings *Low Fat*

2 pounds boneless chicken, cut into strips
1/4 cup chopped green onion (1.8 g)
4 tsp fresh ginger (2 g)
1 g garli

103
Low Carb & No Carb Cookbook. (A) 130-Recipes. (B) 85-Low Carb Desserts. (C) 27-Restaurant Guide To Eating Out.

clove, crushed (0.9 g) 1 tbsp sesame oil 1 tbsp sesam

104
Low Carb & No Carb Cookbook. (A) 130-Recipes. (B) 85-Low Carb Desserts. (C) 27-Restaurant Guide To Eating Out.

esame seeds (1.4 g)
salt & pepper to taste

Mix onions with ginger, garlic & 1 tbsp oil. Drench chicken in oil mix, coat with sesame seeds & stir fry until thoroughly cooked.

Carb Count: Recipe Total 6.1 g, Per Serving: 1.7 g

(90) ZUCCHINI CASSEROLE - 4 Servings *Low Fat*

1/2 cup diced tomatoes (5.8 g)
12 slices bacon, cooked & crumbled
1/4 cup Parmesan cheese
salt &

105

Low Carb & No Carb Cookbook. (A) 130-Recipes. (B) 85-Low Carb Desserts. (C) 27-Restaurant Guide To Eating Out.

pepper
to taste
2 pounds chicken, cooked, cut into pieces
1 cup zucchini, chopped (3.8 g)
Preheat oven to 425 degrees F. Mix tomatoes, bacon, Parmesan, salt & pepper. Layer tomato mixture with chicken in oiled casserole dish. Bake for 30 minutes. Add chopped zucchini to dish & cover with shredded cheese. Bake 30 minutes longer until zucchini is tender crisp.

Carb Count: Recipe Total 9.6 g, Per Serving 2.4 g

(91) MIDEASTERN LEMON CHICKEN - 4 Servings *Low Fat*

4 chicken breasts, cut up
1 tbsp lemon juice (1.3 g)
1/2 cup vinegar
2 tbsp olive oil
1 large cucumber, diced (3 g)
1 tomato

106

Low Carb & No Carb Cookbook. (A) 130-Recipes. (B) 85-Low Carb Desserts. (C) 27-Restaurant Guide To Eating Out.

diced (5.8 g)

4 tsp lemon juice (5.2 g)

1 tbsp o

107
Low Carb & No Carb Cookbook. (A) 130-Recipes. (B) 85-Low Carb Desserts. (C) 27-Restaurant Guide To Eating Out.

live oil 2 tbsp fresh cilantro (1 g) da

108
Low Carb & No Carb Cookbook. (A) 130-Recipes. (B) 85-Low Carb Desserts. (C) 27-Restaurant Guide To Eating Out.

s
h

s
a
l
t

Combine lemon juice with 1/2 cup vinegar & 2 tbsp olive oil. Marinate chicken in lemon/vinegar mix for at least 20 minutes. Combine cucumber, tomato with lemon juice, olive oil, cilantro & salt. Put salad in refrigerator until chicken is ready. Spray non-stick skillet with low fat cooking spray. Cook chicken. Serve with cucumber-tomato salad.

Carb Count: Recipe Total 16.3 g, Per Serving 4.1 g
.
(92) GREEK-STYLE SWORDFISH - 4 Servings
*Low

Fat* 4 swordfish steaks juice of one lemon (2.6 g)
8 ounces can Italian-style stewed tomatoes (10.5 g)
1 cup feta cheese, crumbled
2 tbsp olives, sliced (2 g)

Preheat broiler; pour lemon juice over steaks. Place on rack in broiling pan. Broil 4 min each side or until fish is opaque throughout. Meanwhile, heat stewed

Low Carb & No Carb Cookbook. (A) 130-Recipes. (B) 85-Low Carb Desserts. (C) 27-Restaurant Guide To Eating Out.

tomatoes to boiling over med-hi heat; boil 5 minutes until mix is slightly thickened. Spoon stewed tomatoes onto 4 dinner plates, range swordfish on top, sprinkle with cheese & olives.

Carb Count: Recipe Total 15.1 g, Per Serving 3.8 g

(93) CHICKEN OSSO BUCO STYLE- 4 Servings *Low Fat*

4 chicken breasts, skin & fat removed
1 tsp salt
1/4 cup chopped onion (3.4 g)
1 large carrot (7 g)
1/2 cup celery (1.5 g)
8-ounce Italian-style stewed tomato (10 g)
1 tbsp chopped fresh parsley (0.3 g)

Spray skillet with cooking spray. Over medium-high heat, add chicken & salt. Cook until golden brown on both sides. Transfer to bowl.
Meanwhile, cut onion & dice carrots & celery. Add to skillet & cook onmedium 10 min until lightly browned. Return chicken to skillet; add tomatoes. Heat to boiling over high heat. Reduce heat to low. Cover & simmer 25 minutes or until juices run clear when chicken is pierced.

Carb Count: Recipe Total 22.2 g, Per Serving 5.5 g

(94) INDONESIAN CHICKEN - 4 Servings *Low Fat*

Low Carb & No Carb Cookbook. (A) 130-Recipes. (B) 85-Low Carb Desserts. (C) 27-Restaurant Guide To Eating Out.

1/4 cup green onion, sliced thin (1.6 g)
1 garlic clove, minced (0.9 g)
1 lime (2.8 g)
1 orange (4 g)
2 tbsp soy sauce
1/2 tsp crushed red pepper (0.5 g)
1/2 tsp ground cumin (0.4 g)
4 chicken breast halves
1 tsp cornstarch
1 tbsp fresh cilantro for garnish (0.5 g)

Spray skillet with cooking spray. Add onion & garlic & cook 2-3 minutes.
Transfer to large bowl. Grate peel & squeeze juice from both the lime & the orange. Set aside orange juice. Add all peel & lime juice to bowl with green onion; stir in soy, pepper & cumin. Cut chicken into strips; add to soy mix & coat; cover & marinate 15 min; remove chicken from marinade. Reserve marinade. Spray skillet with cooking spray. Add chicken & cook. In small bowl, mix cornstarch & orange juice. Add to skillet with reserved marinade. Cook until mix thickens. Boil 1 minute.
Return chicken to skillet. Heat through & serve.

Carb Count: Recipe Total 10.7 g, Per Serving 2.6 g

(95) **MARINATED STEAK - 4 Servings**
Low Fat

1
clo

111

Low Carb & No Carb Cookbook. (A) 130-Recipes. (B) 85-Low Carb Desserts. (C) 27-Restaurant Guide To Eating Out.

ve ga rlic , mi nc ed (0.9 g)
1 tsp cu mi n (0.8 g)
large pinch of chili powder (0.7 g)
1 tsp salt
1 tsp black pepper
2 tablespoons red wine
4 sirloin steaks

Combine all ingredients (except the steak) together. Prick the meat all over with fork tines and cover with the marinade in a shallow pan. Refrigerate meat overnight. Drain well before grilling. Grill or broil over medium heat about 15-20 minutes per piece (turning once). Enjoy with sautéed green beans & red peppers.

Carb Count: Recipe Total 2.4 g, Per Serving 0.6 g

Low Carb & No Carb Cookbook. (A) 130-Recipes. (B) 85-Low Carb Desserts. (C) 27-Restaurant Guide To Eating Out.

(96) MOROCCAN CHICKEN STEW - 4 Servings *Low Fat*

4 skinless boneless chicken breasts
2 tsp ground cumin (1.8 g)
2 tsp ginger (2.6 g)
1/8 teaspoon cayenne pepper (0.1 g)
2 1/2 cups chicken broth
1/2 cup shredded zucchini (1.9 g)
salt and black pepper
2 tbsp chopped fresh cilantro (0.5 g)
cornstarch solution, to thicken

Heat a nonstick saucepan. Cut chicken into bite-sized pieces. Add oil to pan. Sauté chicken. Add the cumin, ginger, and cayenne. Cook, stirring.
Add broth, stir and bring just to a boil. Reduce heat, cover and simmer. Add zucchini to the stew. Bring to a boil; reduce heat to simmer uncovered. Heat through & serve.

Carb Count: Recipe Total 6.9 g, Per Serving 1.8 g

113

Low Carb & No Carb Cookbook. (A) 130-Recipes. (B) 85-Low Carb Desserts. (C) 27-Restaurant Guide To Eating Out.

(97) HONEY-LIME GLAZED CHICKEN- 4 Servings *Low Fat*

1/8 cup honey (12 g)
2 tbsp lime juice (2.8 g)
2 tbsp chopped cilantro (0.5 g)
1 tbsp soy sauce
2 tsp jalapeno pepper (0.5 g)
1 tsp minced garlic (0.5 g)
4 skinless boneless chicken breast halves
1 tsp cornstarch
3/4 cup chicken broth

In a glass dish combine the ingredients for the marinade; mix well. Trim the chicken breasts of fat and pound gently to even the thickness. Place the chicken in the marinade; turn to coat both sides. Cover, and let marinate at room temperature for 30 minutes, turning once. Heat a skillet or grill-pan to medium-high. Add cooking spray. Reserving the marinade, add the chicken to the skillet. Cook until chicken is golden brown. Using to the reserved marinade add broth and cornstarch. Mix well. Push the chicken aside and add marinade to pan drippings; stir constantly and deglaze the pan. Add more water as needed. Serve chicken with sauce.

Carb Count: Recipe Total 16.3 g, Per Serving 4 g

(98) FISH WITH BLACK BEANS & SALSA - 3 Servings *Low Fat*

3 white fish fillets
1 tbsp lime juice (1.4 g)
1/4 cup cooked black beans (8 g)
1 large garlic clove, chopped (0.9 g)
1 tsp unsalted butter
1/2 cup diced tomatoes
1/4 cup diced zucchini (0.9 g)
1/2 teaspoon sun-dried tomato paste
(0.2 g) 1/2 cup broth
1 cup shredded romaine lettuce (1.9 g)
2 tbsp soy sauce
1 tbsp malt vinegar
1/8 cup plain yogurt (1.4 g)

Squeeze lime on fish fillets. Salt & pepper to taste. Set aside. In a small nonstick saucepan, warm the beans over medium heat with garlic and butter. Dice and add the tomatoes, zucchini and chipotle pepper with sauce to taste. Add the sun-dried tomato paste, broth and season with western spice blend. Keep warm, add water as needed. Combine soy sauce, malt vinegar, pinch of salt and yogurt. Meanwhile preheat grill. Grill the fish for 2 -3 minutes, or until flaky. To serve cut fish fillets into long fingers and place in the center salad. Top with dressing & serve.

115

Low Carb & No Carb Cookbook. (A) 130-Recipes. (B) 85-Low Carb Desserts. (C) 27-Restaurant Guide To Eating Out.

Carb Count: Recipe Total 14.7 g, Per Serving 4.9 g

(99) SNAPPER WITH LEMON BASIL SAUCE - 2 Servings *Low Fat

2
snapper
or firm
white
fish fillets
salt and
freshly
ground
black
pepper
paprika
1/2 cup finely diced red bell pepper (4 g)
1/4 cup finely diced green onions (1.8 g)
4 tsp chopped fresh basil (3.6 g)
1 tbsp snipped chives (0.6 g)
2 tsp olive oil
1 tsp butter
1 tbsp fresh lemon juice (1.3 g)
2 tbsp white wine vinegar

Divide the fillets into 4 pieces. Sprinkle lightly with salt, pepper and paprika. Set aside and dice the bell pepper and green onions. Place a large non-stick skillet over high heat. When hot, add the oil. Place fish in the pan and fry for 2 minutes; turn gently. Place the thinner pieces toward the rim of the pan, and make room. Add the peppers, onions, basil and chives. Reduce heat, add the lemon juice & white wine vinegar. Serve

.

116

Low Carb & No Carb Cookbook. (A) 130-Recipes. (B) 85-Low Carb Desserts. (C) 27-Restaurant Guide To Eating Out.

Carb Count: Recipe Total 11.3 g, Per Serving 5.6 g

(100) <u>SHRIMP AND GARLIC BUTTER - 4 Servings</u>

1 pound fresh or frozen shrimp
2 tbsp butter
1 clove garlic, minced (0.9 g)
1 tbsp fresh parsley (0.3 g)
1 tbsp dry sherry

Thaw shrimp, if frozen. Peel & devein, rinse & pat dry. Heat butter in skillet. Add shrimp & garlic. Cook for 3 minutes until shrimp turns pink. Stir in parsley & sherry. For variety, use scallops instead of shrimp.

Carb Count: Recipe Total 1.2 g, Per Serving 0.3 g

(101) <u>ORANGE ROUGHY WITH LEMON SAUCE - 2 Servings</u>

117

Low Carb & No Carb Cookbook. (A) 130-Recipes. (B) 85-Low Carb Desserts. (C) 27-Restaurant Guide To Eating Out.

2 orange rough fillets

1/3 cup water

1/4 cup white wine
1 tbsp each parsley (0.3 g) and fresh lemon juice (1.3 g)
1/2 tsp chicken bouillon

Heat oil in skillet. Add fillets and cook over medium high heat turning once, until fish is cooked thoroughly, usually 3-5 minutes on each side. Transfer fish to a platter. To the same skillet add water, wine, parsley, lemon juice, and bouillon. Cook over high heat until mixture comes to a boil; continue to cook until mixture is reduced to about 1/4 cup of, about 4-5 minutes. Pour over fish and serve.

Carb Count: Recipe Total 1.6 g, Per Serving 0.8 g

(102) CRAB LEGS - 4 Servings *Low Fat*

2 pounds fresh or frozen crab legs
8 tbsp butter, melted
2 tsp fresh basil (1 g)
1/2 tsp lemon zest (0.1 g)
1 tbsp lemon juice (1.3 g)

Thaw crab legs, if frozen. Rinse & pat dry with paper towels. Combine butter with basil, lemon zest & lemon juice. Brush crab legs with half of butter mixture & broil in greased pan. Serve with remaining butter mixture.

Carb Count: Recipe Total 2.4 g, Per Serving 0.6 g

119
Low Carb & No Carb Cookbook. (A) 130-Recipes. (B) 85-Low Carb Desserts. (C) 27-Restaurant Guide To Eating Out.

(103) ITALIAN CHICKEN - 4 Servings

1/2 packet Italian Seasoning (4 g carbs)
1/4 cup mayonnaise
1/4 cup water
1/3 cup balsamic vinegar (7 g carbs)
1/2 cup olive oil
2 chicken breasts

Combine all ingredients except chicken. Coat chicken breasts with sauce.
Bake for 40 minutes at 375 degrees.

Carb Count: Recipe Total 11 g, Per Serving 2.7 g

(104) VEGETABLE BEEF SOUP - 4 Servings

3 pounds beef, cut into bit sized pieces
1 garlic clove diced (0.9 g)
1/2 celery rib, diced (0.4 g carbs)
olive oil
3 cups beef broth
1 cup water
1/4 cup red wine
14 oz can diced

120
Low Carb & No Carb Cookbook. (A) 130-Recipes. (B) 85-Low Carb Desserts. (C) 27-Restaurant Guide To Eating Out.

tomato, with juice (14 g)
salt and pepper to taste 1 cup cauliflower (2.6 g carbs)
1/2 cup shredded zucchini (1.9 g carbs)

Heat oil in a large pot. Add beef, garlic and celery. Cook until meat is browned on all sides and onions are translucent. Add the broth, water, tomato, wine and spices. Bring to a boil, then cover and reduce to low heat. Let simmer gently for 1 hour, stirring occasionally. Add cauliflower and zucchini. Bring back to a boil, cover, turn down the heat, and cook until heated through.

Carb Count: Recipe Total 19.8 g, Per Serving 4.9 g

(105) CAULIFLOWER CREAM SOUP

2 cups cauliflower, diced (5 g)
1/2 cup fresh parsley (1.9 g)
1 cup water
3 cups chicken broth
1 cup cream (9.6 g)
1/2 cup water salt and pepper to taste

Heat oil over medium heat. Add cauliflower and parsley. Cover and cook 10 minutes more. Add water and broth and bring to a boil. Cover and simmer 5 minutes. Add cream, salt & pepper. Heat & serve.

121
Low Carb & No Carb Cookbook. (A) 130-Recipes. (B) 85-Low Carb Desserts. (C) 27-Restaurant Guide To Eating Out.

Carb Count: Recipe Total 16.9 g, Per Serving 4.2 g

(106) <u>CLAM CHOWDER - 4 Servings</u>

3 slices bacon, cut into small pieces, cooked
6-ounce can chopped clams, with juice
1 cup water
1 cup cream (9.6 g)
Salt and pepper to taste

Cook bacon. Add the clams and water. Cover and simmer for about 15-20 minutes. Turn off the heat and add the cream, salt and pepper.

Carb Count: Recipe Total 9.6 g, Per Serving 2.4 g

(107) <u>SAUSAGE SOUP - 4 Servings</u>

1 pound ground sausage
3 slices bacon
1 cup cream (9.6 g)
1 cup fresh s

122
Low Carb & No Carb Cookbook. (A) 130-Recipes. (B) 85-Low Carb Desserts. (C) 27-Restaurant Guide To Eating Out.

pinach (2.4 g) 4 cups chicken broth

Garlic, salt, pepper to taste

123
Low Carb & No Carb Cookbook. (A) 130-Recipes. (B) 85-Low Carb Desserts. (C) 27-Restaurant Guide To Eating Out.

Steam cauliflower until soft. Cook sausage and bacon. Place all ingredients in a large pot. Bring to a boil. Reduce heat & simmer for 20 minutes.

Carb Count: Recipe Total 17 g, Per Serving 4.2 g

(108) GRILLED STEAK - 4 Servings

2 pounds steak
2 tbsp butter
2 tsp Worcestershire sauce

Combine butter and Worcestershire sauce. Dip meat in butter mix and grill. Serve with herbed butter (combine butter 1 tbsp fresh parsley (0.3 g), or 1 tbsp fresh chopped chives (0.6 g), or 1 clove minced garlic (0.9 g), or 3 tsp fresh rosemary (2.4 g), or 3 tsp fresh basil (2.7 g).

Carb Count: Recipe Total 0 g, Per Serving 0 g

(109) STEAK AND BACON - 4 Servings

4 slices bacon
2 pounds steak
1/2 cup sour cream (8 g; check your brand)
3 tbsp chives (1.8 g)

Cook bacon. Grill steaks. Combine sour cream with chives. Serve steak with sour cream. Crumble bacon and sprinkle over the top.

Low Carb & No Carb Cookbook. (A) 130-Recipes. (B) 85-Low Carb Desserts. (C) 27-Restaurant Guide To Eating Out.

Carb Count: Recipe Total 9.8 g, Per Serving 2.9 g

(110) GRILLED ROSEMARY CHICKEN - 4 Servings

4 chicken breasts
2 tbsp olive oil
2 cloves garlic, crushed (1.8 g)
4 tbsp fresh rosemary, crushed (3.2 g)
2 tsp fresh thyme, crushed (2 g)

Mix oil, garlic, rosemary & thyme. Drench chicken in marinade. Grill.

Carb Count: Recipe Total 7 g, Per Serving 1.8 g

(111) HOT PEPPER CHICKEN - 4 Servings

4 chicken breasts, cut into strips
2 tbsp olive oil
2 tbsp hot pepper sauce
salt and pepper

Combine oil with hot pepper sauce, salt & pepper. Drench chicken in sauce. Grill or broil.

Carb Count: Recipe Total 0 g, Per Serving 0 g

(112) ROASTED CHICKEN WITH BACON - 4 Serving *Low Fat*

125
Low Carb & No Carb Cookbook. (A) 130-Recipes. (B) 85-Low Carb Desserts. (C) 27-Restaurant Guide To Eating Out.

4 boneless skinless chicken breasts
4 slices bacon
2 tsp garlic powder (4 g)
1 cup grated cauliflower (4.4 g)

Place the cauliflower in a greased pan. Place chicken breasts on top of cauliflower and sprinkle with garlic powder. Place bacon over chicken and bake for an hour at 350 degrees F until the bacon is crispy.

Carb Count: Recipe Total 8.4 g, Per Serving 4.2 g

(113) <u>LEMON ROASTED CHICKEN - 4 Servings *Low Fat*</u>

1 whole chicken salt

126
Low Carb & No Carb Cookbook. (A) 130-Recipes. (B) 85-Low Carb Desserts. (C) 27-Restaurant Guide To Eating Out.

& pepper
1 tsp oregano
1 clove garlic, minced (0.9 g)
2 tbsp butter, melted 1 cup chicken broth
2 tbsp lemon juice (2.6 g)

Remove the giblets and neck, wash the chicken and pat it dry. Salt & pepper the chicken to taste. Place in roasting pan. Sprinkle half the Oregano and Garlic inside the cavity, and half outside. Add butter and chicken broth. Cover and roast at 350 degrees F for 1 - 1 1/2 hours.

Low Carb & No Carb Cookbook. (A) 130-Recipes. (B) 85-Low Carb Desserts. (C) 27-Restaurant Guide To Eating Out.

During the 30 minutes of cooking add the lemon juice.

Carb Count: Recipe Total 3.5 g, Per Serving 0.9 g

(114) <u>SAUSAGE STUFFED CHICKEN - 4 Servings</u>

1 pound pork sausage
1/8 cup fresh parsley, chopped (0.3 g)
1 garlic clove, minced (0.9 g)1/2 tsp thyme (0.5 g)
1/2 tsp salt
1 egg, beaten
1/2 tsp pepper
1/2 tsp sage (0.2 g)
4 chicken breasts, flattened

Brown sausage in a large frying pan, breaking up with a fork. When all the pink is gone and sausage is thoroughly cooked, remove from heat.
Drain excess fat from sausage meat.
Add remaining ingredients and mix well.
Place on flattened chicken breasts, roll up, and secure with a toothpick. Bake at 425 degrees F for 35-40 minutes.

Carb Count: Recipe Total 1.9 g, Per Serving 0.5 g

(115) <u>ORANGE CHICKEN - 2 Servings *Low Fat*</u>

1 pound boneless chicken, cut up

128

Low Carb & No Carb Cookbook. (A) 130-Recipes. (B) 85-Low Carb Desserts. (C) 27-Restaurant Guide To Eating Out.

4 tbsp butter

1 tsp orange zest (0.5

129

Low Carb & No Carb Cookbook. (A) 130-Recipes. (B) 85-Low Carb Desserts. (C) 27-Restaurant Guide To Eating Out.

g
)

salt & pepper

Melt butter, stir in orange zest. Drench chicken in butter mix & stir fry until cooked thoroughly.
Optional, use lemon zest (0.3 g per teaspoon)

Carb Count: Recipe Total 0.5 g, Per Serving 0.25 g

(116) ASPARAGUS CHICKEN - 3 Servings
*Low

Fat* salt & pepper 3 large chicken breasts 2 tbsp butter
1 pound asparagus (8.8 g)
1/2 cup chicken broth
2 tsp cornstarch

Salt & pepper chicken. Melt butter in skillet. Add chicken & cook. Remove. Add asparagus & 1/4 cup water. Heat to boiling. Reduce heat & simmer for 5 minutes. Mix chicken broth with 2 tsp cornstarch until smooth. Add to asparagus. Heat to boiling. Boil 1 minute. Reduce heat. Return chicken to pan. Heat & serve.

Carb Count: Recipe Total 8.8 g, Per Serving 2.9 g

130

Low Carb & No Carb Cookbook. (A) 130-Recipes. (B) 85-Low Carb Desserts. (C) 27-Restaurant Guide To Eating Out.

(117) MOROCCAN CHICKEN - 4 Servings
Low Fat

1 pound boneless chicken, cut up
1 tbsp butter
1 tsp cumin (0.9 g)
1/2 tsp cinn

131

Low Carb & No Carb Cookbook. (A) 130-Recipes. (B) 85-Low Carb Desserts. (C) 27-Restaurant Guide To Eating Out.

a mon (0.9g) salt & pepper to taste

132

Low Carb & No Carb Cookbook. (A) 130-Recipes. (B) 85-Low Carb Desserts. (C) 27-Restaurant Guide To Eating Out.

7 ounces can tomatoes, drained & chopped (7 g)
1 tbsp fresh cilantro, chopped (1 g)

Melt butter in pan. Add chicken and spices. Cook for 5 minutes. Add tomatoes. Bring to boiling. Reduce heat; cover & simmer for 15 minutes.
Carb Count: Recipe Total 9.8 g, Per Serving 2.4 g

(118) CHICKEN CORDON BLEU - 4 Servings

4 boneless skinless chicken breasts
4 slices of ham
Swiss cheese slices
1

133
Low Carb & No Carb Cookbook. (A) 130-Recipes. (B) 85-Low Carb Desserts. (C) 27-Restaurant Guide To Eating Out.

t b s p melted butter

1 egg; beaten

1 cup Parmesan cheese

Flatten chicken. Roll up with ham & cheese; secure with a toothpick. Combine egg & butter. Dip chicken in butter & then cheese.

134

Low Carb & No Carb Cookbook. (A) 130-Recipes. (B) 85-Low Carb Desserts. (C) 27-Restaurant Guide To Eating Out.

Place in greased baking dish. Bake at 350" F for about 35 minutes or until golden brown.

Carb Count: Recipe Total 0 g, Per Serving 0 g

(119) TERIYAKI FISH STEAKS - 4 Servings *Low Fat*

1 pound fresh or frozen tuna or halibut steaks
1/2 cup soy sauce
2 tbsp orange juice (2 g)
1 tbsp oil
1 tbsp dry sherry
1/4 tsp ginger (0.3 g)

135
Low Carb & No Carb Cookbook. (A) 130-Recipes. (B) 85-Low Carb Desserts. (C) 27-Restaurant Guide To Eating Out.

1 tsp honey (3 g)

1 clove garlic, minced (0.9 g)

Combine all ingredients except fish. Pour marinade over fish. Let sit for 30 minutes-2 hours. Drain fish, reserving marinade. Broil fish for 5 minutes. Baste with sauce & Broil on other side for 5 minutes.

Carb Count: Recipe Total 6.2 g, Per Serving 1.5 g

(120) SAUSAGE IN GRAVY - 4 servings

1 1/2 pounds smoked sausage, cut into pieces
6 1/2 cups beef broth
1/4 cup chopped celery (1 g)
1/4 cup green peppers, chopped (1.6 g)

Low Carb & No Carb Cookbook. (A) 130-Recipes. (B) 85-Low Carb Desserts. (C) 27-Restaurant Guide To Eating Out.

1 clove garlic, minced (0.9 g)
2 tbsp tomato sauce (0.8 g)
4 tbsp parsley (1.2 g)
1/3 cup green onions, diced (2.2 g)
1 tsp cayenne pepper (1 g)

Melt butter in large skillet. Add sausage, cover, and cook without stirring about 10 minutes. Add 3/4 cup of stock and scrape bottom. Add salt and pepper. Cover and cook 2 minutes. Add celery, green peppers and garlic. Cover and cook 3 minutes, scraping bottom of pan. Add tomato sauce and cook uncovered 10 minutes, scraping occasionally. Add parsley and green onions. Add 3 1/4 cup of more stock and scrape. Cook 20 minutes
until liquid is thick dark red gravy. Stir occasionally. Stir in remaining stock. Bring to boil, reduce heat, and simmer, stirring frequently, about 14 minutes, until gravy is right consistency. Remove from heat and serve immediately.

Carb Count: Recipe Total 8.7 g, Per Serving 2.2 g

(121) CHEESY MEATLOAF - 8 servings

2 pounds ground beef
1/4 cup chopped onion (3.4 g)
2 eggs, eaten
1
/
2

c

137

Low Carb & No Carb Cookbook. (A) 130-Recipes. (B) 85-Low Carb Desserts. (C) 27-Restaurant Guide To Eating Out.

up cream (4.8g) 1/2 cup water salt & p

138

Low Carb & No Carb Cookbook. (A) 130-Recipes. (B) 85-Low Carb Desserts. (C) 27-Restaurant Guide To Eating Out.

e
p
p
e
r

garlic salt
1 1/2 c mozzarella cheese
12 oz can tomato sauce (15 g)
Combine ground beef, onion, eggs, cream, salt, pepper and garlic salt in large bowl. Mix well. Add more cream, if dry. Turn onto long piece of waxed paper. Pat mixture into rectangle. Spread mozzarella cheese over mixture. Start from one end and lift waxed paper and roll mixture into a log shape. Carefully, place in large oven-proof casserole dish, seam down. Pinch ends to seal. Pour tomato sauce over mixture. Bake at 375 degrees F for 1 to 1 1/2 hours or until done.

Carb Count: Recipe Total 23.2 g, Per Serving 2.9 g

(122) CREAMY PORK CHOPS - 6 servings

6

p
o
r
k

c
h
o
p
s

139
Low Carb & No Carb Cookbook. (A) 130-Recipes. (B) 85-Low Carb Desserts. (C) 27-Restaurant Guide To Eating Out.

salt & pepper 1 tsp paprika (1.2 g) but

140
Low Carb & No Carb Cookbook. (A) 130-Recipes. (B) 85-Low Carb Desserts. (C) 27-Restaurant Guide To Eating Out.

ter to fry in 3/4 cup light cream (3.6

141
Low Carb & No Carb Cookbook. (A) 130-Recipes. (B) 85-Low Carb Desserts. (C) 27-Restaurant Guide To Eating Out.

8 oz cream cheese)

1/2 cup Parmesan cheese

Preheat oven to 350 degrees F. Season the chops and brown in butter. Heat cream. Add cream cheese and 1/4 cup of Parmesan cheese, mixing until blended. Place chops in baking dish. Cover with sauce, and remaining Parmesan cheese. Bake for 50 minutes.

Carb Count: Recipe Total 4.8 g, Per Serving 0.8 g

(123) STUFFED CABBAGE - 4 servings

1 whole cabbage (12 g)

142

Low Carb & No Carb Cookbook. (A) 130-Recipes. (B) 85-Low Carb Desserts. (C) 27-Restaurant Guide To Eating Out.

1/2 cup spinach, cooked (3.2 g)
1 tbsp fresh parsley, chopped (0.3 g)
1 pound ground beef, cooked
1
/
2

c
u
p

P
a
r
m
e
s
a
n

c
h
e
e
s
e

2

e
g
g
s
,
b
e
a

143
Low Carb & No Carb Cookbook. (A) 130-Recipes. (B) 85-Low Carb Desserts. (C) 27-Restaurant Guide To Eating Out.

t
e
n

salt and pepper

Rinse cabbage. Boil whole in salted water for 5 minutes. Drain well. Combine spinach, parsley, beef, cheese & eggs. Remove leaves from cabbage & stuff with ground beef mixture. Place in baking dish and cover with 4 tbsp oil. Bake for 25 minutes at 350 degrees F or until cabbage is tender. For less carbs, simply shred cabbage & heat in skillet with ground beef mixture (1 c cooked cabbage is 6.2 g)

Carb Count: Recipe Total 15.5 g, Per Serving 4.8 g

(124) CILANTRO CHICKEN - 4 Servings *Low Fat*

2 boneless chicken breasts
2

t
b
s
p

l
i
m
e

j

144

Low Carb & No Carb Cookbook. (A) 130-Recipes. (B) 85-Low Carb Desserts. (C) 27-Restaurant Guide To Eating Out.

uice (2.6g) 2 tbsp white wine 1 tbsp

145
Low Carb & No Carb Cookbook. (A) 130-Recipes. (B) 85-Low Carb Desserts. (C) 27-Restaurant Guide To Eating Out.

s
o
y

s
a
u
c
e

1 clove garlic (0.9 g)
1 tbsp. chopped fresh cilantro (0.3 g)
1/2 tsp chili powder (0.7 g)

Rinse chicken and pat dry. Arrange in a shallow dish. Combine remaining ingredients. Pour over chicken. Cover. Refrigerate 2 to 3 hours. Turn occasionally. Spray grill with non-stick cooking spray. Grill 7 to 9 minutes on each side. Baste while grilling.

Carb Count: Recipe Total 4.5 g, Per Serving 1.1 g

(125) BRAISED TUNA - 4 Servings *Low Fat*

4 Tuna Filets
2 tbsp oil
1/2 cup sliced celery (1.9 g)
1/2 cup tomato, chopped (5.8 g)
1/2 tsp thyme (0.5 g)
1 1/4 cup white wine

Heat 1 tablespoon of the oil and stir fry the celery until soft. Stir in tomatoes and thyme

146
Low Carb & No Carb Cookbook. (A) 130-Recipes. (B) 85-Low Carb Desserts. (C) 27-Restaurant Guide To Eating Out.

and cook for about 5 minutes. Place in shallow dish.
Heat remaining oil and quickly fry the tuna steaks to brown on each side.
Place tuna steaks on top of vegetables, season; then pour over white wine. Cover. Bake at 325" F for 40-50 minutes until fish is tender.

Carb Count: Recipe Total 8.2 g, Per Serving 4 g

(126) BEEF CURRY - 4 Servings *Low Fat*

1 1/2 pounds steak, cut into cubes 4 tbsp olive oil
2 cloves garlic, minced (1.8 g)
2 tsp minced fresh ginger (2.6 g)
1 tsp ground coriander (0.5 g)
1 tsp ground cumin (0.9 g)
1/4 tsp dried red pepper flakes (0.2 g)
1/2 tsp salt
2 tablespoons water
3 tablespoons chopped cilantro (0.9 g)

147
Low Carb & No Carb Cookbook. (A) 130-Recipes. (B) 85-Low Carb Desserts. (C) 27-Restaurant Guide To Eating Out.

In a large frying pan, heat the oil over moderate heat. Add the garlic and ginger and cook, stirring, for 1 minute. Meanwhile, in a small bowl, combine the coriander, cumin, red-pepper flakes, salt, and water. Add to the garlic and cook, stirring, for 1 minute. Add the meat to the pan and cook, stirring, for 3 minutes. Raise the heat to moderately high and cook thoroughly. Remove from heat. Stir in the cilantro.

Carb Count: Recipe Total 6 g, Per Serving 1.5 g

(127) **PORK CHOPS & APPLESAUCE - 4 Servings**

4 pork chops
1/4 cup white wine 8 ounces unsweetened applesauce (18 g; check your brand)

Preheat oven to 350 degrees F. In a skillet, brown chops in butter.
Place in casserole dish. Combine wine & applesauce & pour over chops.
Bake for 1 hour.
Carb Count: Recipe Total 18 g, Per Serving 4.5 g

(128) **LOW CARB CHILI - 4 Servings**

4 slices bacon
1 pound hamburger
2 cloves garlic, chopped fine (1.8 g)
1/2 cup of green bell pepper, diced (3.2 g)
1 tsp cumin (0.9 g)

148
Low Carb & No Carb Cookbook. (A) 130-Recipes. (B) 85-Low Carb Desserts. (C) 27-Restaurant Guide To Eating Out.

2 tsp chili powder (2.8 g) 2 tsp hot pepper sauce
1 tbsp Worcestershire sauce
14 ounce canned tomatoes, with juice (14 g)

Cook the bacon until crisp in a large pot, then remove bacon. Sauté the hamburger in the drippings. Add garlic, green pepper, cumin, and chili powder. Add remaining ingredients. Crumble bacon & return with the hamburger to the pot. Simmer for 25 minutes.
Carb Count: Recipe Total 22.7 g, Per Serving 5.6 g

(129) STUFFED SAUSAGE - 6 Servings

2 tbsp chopped parsley (0.6 g)
1 tbsp chopped chives (0.6 g)
1 cup cream cheese
2 pounds sausage
salt & pepper

Pre- heat oven to 400 degrees F. Mix parsley, chives & cream cheese & roll into 12 small balls. Wrap sausage around each ball. Bake for 35-40 minutes.

Carb Count: Recipe Total 1.2 g, Per Serving 0.2 g

(130) STUFFED EGGPLANT - 4 Servings

1 egg plant
1 tsp chili powder (1.4 g)

149
Low Carb & No Carb Cookbook. (A) 130-Recipes. (B) 85-Low Carb Desserts. (C) 27-Restaurant Guide To Eating Out.

1 garlic clove, minced (0.9 g)
1 tsp salt
1/2 cup tomato, chopped (5.8 g)
1 pound ground turkey
1 red bell pepper, chopped (8 g)
1 tbsp fresh cilantro (0.3 g)

Cut eggplant in half & cut out flesh. Place eggplant shells in greased casserole dish. In skillet, heat oil. Add garlic, chili powder & salt. Add tomato & cook for 5 minutes. Add ground turkey to skillet & cook for 10 more minutes. Add bell pepper & cook a few more

150
Low Carb & No Carb Cookbook. (A) 130-Recipes. (B) 85-Low Carb Desserts. (C) 27-Restaurant Guide To Eating Out.

minutes. Spoon the turkey into the eggplant shells & brush edges with oil. Bake at 350 degrees for 20-25 minutes.

Carb Count: Recipe Total 8.4 g, Per Serving 2.1 g

INDEX
****

BREAKFAST
1. CRUSTLESS QUICHE 1.9 g
2. MOCK FRENCH TOAST 1.6 g
3. LOW CARB WAFFLES 3.3 g
4. ZUCCHINI HASH BROWNS 1.9 g
5. BACON CHEESE MUFFINS 4.8 g
6. CHEESE BLINTZES 5.8 g
7. COTTAGE SCRAMBLED EGGS 3.7 g
8. APPLE & BRIE EGGS 2.8 g
9. LOW CARB PANCAKES 1.8 g
10. FRITTATA 2.5 g
11. SOUTHWEST QUICHE 3.2 g
12. BACON BREAKFAST PIE 3.5 g
13. HAM & CHEESE OMELET 0.2 g
14. SCRAMBLED EGG PIZZA 1.2 g
15. SAUSAGE OR BACON BURRITO 3.7 g
16. FAJITA BREAKFAST BURRITO 5 g
17. PEACHES & RICOTTA 2.9 g
18. PUFFED OVEN PANCAKE 2.5 g

151
Low Carb & No Carb Cookbook. (A) 130-Recipes. (B) 85-Low Carb Desserts. (C) 27-Restaurant Guide To Eating Out.

19. CREPES 5 g
20. EGGS BENEDICT 0.3 g
21. DENVER SCRAMBLED EGGS 1.7 g
22. PUFFY OMELET WITH CHEESE SAUCE 1.6 g
23. OVEN OMELET 0 g
24. APRICOT SOUFFLES 4.5 g
25. APPLE SAUSAGE PATTIES 2.7 g
26. SPINACH PUFFS 1.5 g
27. RASPBERRY CREAM 4.5 g
28. BLACKBERRY SYRUP 2.3 g
29. MAPLE BUTTER 0 g
30. MAPLE SYRUP 0 g

LUNCH

31. CHEF SALAD 1.7 g
32. BLACKENED CHICKEN SALAD 2.7 g
33. COBB SALAD 0.8 g
34. TURKEY & CRANBERRY SALAD 4.2 g
35. CHICKEN NAAN 2 g
36. CHINESE CHICKEN SALAD 1.4 g
37. BLT SALAD 3.7 g
38. TURKEY & CREAM CHEESE 2 g
39. ITALIAN MEAT & CHEESE 4.2 g
40. FETA SPINACH SALAD 2.6 g
41. ROAST BEEF & CHEESE 3.5 g
42. SPINACH WITH CHICKEN & APRICOTS 3.7 g
43. BUFFALO CHICKEN WINGS 0 g
44. TUNA MELT 3.9 g
45. CHICKEN & PROVOLONE SALAD 1.4 g
46. SMOKED SALMON MUFFINS 5.5 g
47. BEEF MINESTRONE 5.1 g
48. BEEF JERKY 0.6 g

152

Low Carb & No Carb Cookbook. (A) 130-Recipes. (B) 85-Low Carb Desserts. (C) 27-Restaurant Guide To Eating Out.

- 49. WALDORF CHICKEN SALAD 3.8 g
- 50. SEAFOOD SALAD 2 g
- 51. SALMON PATTIES 1 g
- 52. ZUCCHINI BOATS 2.6 g
- 53. STUFFED MUSHROOMS 2.2 g
- 54. SALMON AND CUCUMBER 2 g
- 55. TUNA SPREAD 1.5 g
- 56. CHILI CHEESE BURGERS 1.2 g
- 57. GOAT CHEESE WITH SPINACH 1.1 g
- 58. SOUTHWEST HAMBURGER 1.5 g
- 59. CHILI CHEESE HOT DOGS 2.9 g
- 60. HAMBURGER PIZZA 2.9 g

DINNER

- 61. GRILLED SESAME SALMON 3.3 g
- 62. CHICKEN PARMESAN 2.5 g
- 63. CHICKEN WITH PEANUT SAUCE 3 g
- 64. CHICKEN TIKKA SALAD 4 g
- 65. MARSALA CHICKEN 2 g
- 66. MUSTARD CHICKEN 4.1 g
- 67. SLOPPY JOES 1.7 g
- 68. POT ROAST 0 g
- 69. BACON-CHICKEN ROLLS 1.8 g
- 70. STUFFED GREEN PEPPERS 5.8 g
- 71. MEDITERRANEAN CHICKEN 4.7 g
- 72. PEACH GLAZED PORK 1.4 g
- 73. CHICKEN WITH OLIVES 1.4 g
- 74. ARTICHOKE SOUP 5 g
- 75. GREEK CHICKEN 2.5 g
- 76. TURKEY WITH BACON 0.8 g
- 77. TERIYAKI BEEF 1.7 g
- 78. DIJON PORK WITH GRAPES 5.1 g
- 79. BBQ CHICKEN 2.2 g
- 80. CARIBBEAN CHICKEN KABOBS 1.3 g
- 81. TUSCAN CHICKEN CASSEROLE 5.8 g

153

Low Carb & No Carb Cookbook. (A) 130-Recipes. (B) 85-Low Carb Desserts. (C) 27-Restaurant Guide To Eating Out.

82. THAI CHICKEN STIR FRY 3.4 g
83. ORANGE BEEF STIR FRY 3.1 g
84. LEMON FISH 1.6 g
85. CHICKEN WITH SUNDRIED TOMATOES 0.7 g
86. CHICKEN STUFFED WITH BACON 0.5 g
87. CHICKEN STUFFED WITH PROSCIUTTO 0.1 g
88. STUFFED TURKEY ROLLS 1.1 g
89. GRILLED SESAME CHICKEN 1.7 g
90. ZUCCHINI CASSEROLE 2.4 g
91. MIDEASTERN LEMON CHICKEN 4.1 g
92. GREEK-STYLE SWORDFISH 3.8 g
93. CHICKEN OSSO BUCO STYLE 5.5 g
94. INDONESIAN CHICKEN 2.6 g
95. MARINATED STEAK 0.6 g
96. MOROCCAN CHICKEN STEW 1.8 g
97. HONEY-LIME GLAZED CHICKEN 4 g
98. FISH WITH BLACK BEANS & SALSA 4.9 g
99. SNAPPER WITH LEMON BASIL SAUCE 5.6 g
100. SHRIMP AND GARLIC BUTTER 0.3 g
101. ORANGE ROUGHY WITH LEMON SAUCE 0.8 g
102. CRAB LEGS 0.6 g
103. ITALIAN CHICKEN 2.7 g
104. 104. VEGETABLE BEEF SOUP 4.9 g
105. CAULIFLOWER CREAM SOUP 4.2 g
106. CLAM CHOWDER 2.4 g
107. 107. SAUSAGE SOUP 4.2 g
108. 108. GRILLED STEAK 0 g

154

Low Carb & No Carb Cookbook. (A) 130-Recipes. (B) 85-Low Carb Desserts. (C) 27-Restaurant Guide To Eating Out.

109. STEAK AND BACON 2.9 g
110. GRILLED ROSEMARY CHICKEN 1.8 g
111. 111. HOT PEPPER CHICKEN 0 g
112. ROASTED CHICKEN WITH BACON 4.2 g
113. LEMON ROASTED CHICKEN 0.9 g
114. SAUSAGE STUFFED CHICKEN 0.5 g
115. ORANGE CHICKEN 0.2 g
116. ASPARAGUS CHICKEN 2.9 g
117. MOROCCAN CHICKEN 2.4 g
118. CHICKEN CORDON BLEU 0 g
119. TERIYAKI FISH STEAKS 1.2 g
120. SAUSAGE IN GRAVY 2.2 g
121. CHEES

155
Low Carb & No Carb Cookbook. (A) 130-Recipes. (B) 85-Low Carb Desserts. (C) 27-Restaurant Guide To Eating Out.

Y MEATLOAF 2.9 g
122. CREAMY PORK CHOPS 0.8 g
123. STUFFED CABBAGE 4.8 g
124. CILANTRO CHICKEN 1.1 g
125. BRAISED TUNA 4 g
126. BEEF CURRY 1.5 g
127. PORK CHOPS & APPLESAUCE 4.5 g
128. LOW CARB CHILI 5.6 g
129. STUFFED SAUSAGE 0.2 g
130. STUFFED EGGPLANT 2.1 g

85 LOW CARB DESSERTS

****

156
Low Carb & No Carb Cookbook. (A) 130-Recipes. (B) 85-Low Carb Desserts. (C) 27-Restaurant Guide To Eating Out.

Note: These recipes call for Splenda for sweetener. You may substitute whatever sweetener you choose. However, you may be interested to know that The Atkins Center has done research that indicates sweeteners that contain aspartame (such as NutraSweet and Equal) stimulate insulin production (leading to unstable blood sugar, irritability and carbohydrate cravings). Sweeteners that use sucralose (marketed as Splenda) and saccharin (such as Sweet' n Low) have not been shown to stimulate insulin production.
****
****

(1) PECAN MERINGUES - 5 Servings

3 egg whites
1 cup Splenda (24 grams)
1 tbsp chopped pecans (0.6 grams)

Preheat oven to 325 degrees F. Whisk egg whites until stiff. Whisk in Splenda gradually. Beat until meringue is thick. Drop spoonfuls of batter onto greased cookie sheets. Sprinkle with walnuts and bake for 30 minutes. Cool and serve with cream cheese. Makes 30 cookies

Carb Count: Recipe Total 24.6 grams, Per Serving 4.9 grams

(2) LEMON MOUSSE - 4 Servings

4 egg yolks

157

Low Carb & No Carb Cookbook. (A) 130-Recipes. (B) 85-Low Carb Desserts. (C) 27-Restaurant Guide To Eating Out.

1/2 cup Splenda (12 grams)
grated zest and juice of 1 lemon (3 grams)
4 egg whites, room temp
1/2 cup heavy cream (4.6 grams)

Place yolks, Splenda, rind and juice in a double boiler over simmering water. Whisk constantly for 10 minutes until thick. Remove from heat & refrigerate for 30 minutes. Beat cream until stiff. In another bowl, beat egg whites until stiff. Fold lemon mixture into cream and then egg whites into cream. Spoon into glasses & chill.

Carb Count: Recipe Total 19.6 grams, Per Serving 4.9 grams

(3) <u>PINA COLADA ICEE - 4 Servings</u>

2 cup light cream (9.6 grams)
1/2 cup crushed pineapples with juice (12.5 grams)
2 scoops vanilla protein powder
1/2 tsp coconut extract, optional
1 cup crushed ice

Mix all the ingredients in a blender on high. Try with pineapples, peaches or strawberries.

Carb Count: Recipe Total 22.1 grams, Per Serving 5.5 grams

158

Low Carb & No Carb Cookbook. (A) 130-Recipes. (B) 85-Low Carb Desserts. (C) 27-Restaurant Guide To Eating Out.

(4) <u>VANILLA ALMOND MOUSSE - 4 Servings</u>

2 egg whites
1/4 cup Splenda, or to taste
1 1/2 cup cream (14.5 grams)
1/2 cup water
2 tsp vanilla (3 grams)
2 tsp almond extract

Beat two egg whites to soft peaks. Gradually beat in 2 tbsp of Splenda.

Continue to beat to still peaks and set aside. Whip cream until frothy. Gradually beat in remaining Splenda until stiff. Add vanilla and almond extract and mix well. Divide equally among individual cups.

Then cover and freeze.

Carb Count: Recipe Total 17.5 grams, Per Serving 4.3 grams

(5) <u>CHOCOLATE RASPBERRY BROWNIES - 12 Servings</u>

1 cup Splenda (24 grams)
3/4 cup unsweetened cocoa powder (33 grams)
6 eggs
1/4 cup sugar free raspberry preserves (or apricot, or cherry) (18 grams; check your brand)

159
Low Carb & No Carb Cookbook. (A) 130-Recipes. (B) 85-Low Carb Desserts. (C) 27-Restaurant Guide To Eating Out.

1 tsp vanilla (1.5 grams)

1/2 tsp salt

160

Low Carb & No Carb Cookbook. (A) 130-Recipes. (B) 85-Low Carb Desserts. (C) 27-Restaurant Guide To Eating Out.

t

1/2 tsp baking soda
1/4 tsp almond extract
1 cup high gluten flour (24 grams)

Grease a 9x13 inch pan. Set aside. Combine Splenda and cocoa. Gradually add eggs and preserves, beating on low-speed with electric mixer. Add vanilla, salt, and almond extract and beat briefly to mix. Combine flour and baking soda and stir in with a spatula. Do not over mix. Turn into prepared pan. Bake at 325 degree F for 30-35 minutes.
Brownies should be slightly under-baked but not runny in the center.
Allow to cool and cut into small squares.

Carb Count: Recipe Total 100.5 grams, Per Serving 8.3 grams

(6) <u>VANILLA ALMOND COOKIES - 2 Servings</u>

4 egg whites
8 tbsp powdered milk (10 grams)
1 tsp each vanilla & almond extract (1.5 grams)
1/8 cup Splenda (3 grams)

Beat egg whites until stiff. Add skim milk powder. Mix well. Add extracts and sweetener. Spoon drop onto cookie sheet. Bake at 275ᵉF for 45 minutes. Remove from sheet and dust with cinnamon.

161
Low Carb & No Carb Cookbook. (A) 130-Recipes. (B) 85-Low Carb Desserts. (C) 27-Restaurant Guide To Eating Out.

Carb Count: Recipe Total 14.5 grams, Per Serving 7.25 grams

(7) <u>CHOCOLATE ANGEL FOOD CAKE - 10 Servings</u>

1/4 cup flour (22 grams)2 tbsp cocoa (2.5 grams)
2 tbsp cornstarch
5 egg white

162

Low Carb & No Carb Cookbook. (A) 130-Recipes. (B) 85-Low Carb Desserts. (C) 27-Restaurant Guide To Eating Out.

s

1/2 tsp cream tartar
1/2 cup Splenda (12 grams)

Preheat oven to 350 degrees F. Sift flour, cocoa, cornstarch. In a separate bowl, beat egg whites until foamy. Add cream of tartar and whisk until soft peaks form. Add Splenda to egg whites and whisk until blended. Fold in cocoa/flour mix. Spoon into a greased ring mold. Bake for 35 minutes. Turn upside down and allow to cool.

Carb Count: Recipe Total 36.5 grams, Per Serving 3.65 grams

(8) <u>KEY LIME PIE - 4 Servings</u>

1 packet unflavored gelatin
3 tbsp lime juice (4.2 grams)
1/2 cup boiling water
1/2 cup Splenda (12 grams)

163
Low Carb & No Carb Cookbook. (A) 130-Recipes. (B) 85-Low Carb Desserts. (C) 27-Restaurant Guide To Eating Out.

1 cup light cream (4.5 grams) 1 tsp vanilla (1.5 grams)
2 drops green food coloring

Sprinkle gelatin over lime juice and let it stand for 1 minute. Add boiling water and sweetener to gelatin mixture and stir until gelatin is dissolved. Refrigerate about 45 minutes or until slightly thickened. Combine cream and vanilla and freeze 30 minutes. Remove from freezer and whip at high speed until stiff. Spoon pie filling into crust. Chill until firm.

Carb Count: Recipe Total 22.2 grams, Per Serving 5.5 grams

(9) **LOW-CARB FUDGE - 8 Servings**

1 packet unflavored gelatin
1/4 cup water
1 square unsweetened chocolate (4 grams)
1/8 tsp cinnamon (0.2 grams)
1/2 cup Splenda (12 grams)
1/4 cup

water
1/2 cup light cream (2.4 grams)
1/2 tsp vanilla (0.7 grams)

Soften gelatin in 1/4 cup water for 5 minutes. Melt chocolate with cinnamon and sweetener; add milk and water slowly. Add gelatin. Stir until dissolved. Remove from fire. Add vanilla, cool. When mixture begins to thicken, turn into cold pan. When firm cut into pieces.

Carb Count: Recipe Total 19.3 grams, Per Serving 2.4 grams

(10) CREAMY RASPBERRY JELLO - 2 servings

One package sugar free raspberry gelatin
2 cup whipped cream (6.6 grams)

Prepare gelatin according to package directions. Chill 4-6 hours before serving. Remove gelatin and beat thoroughly. Add whipped cream and beat until smooth. Chill & serve.
Carb Count: Recipe Total 6.6 grams, Per Serving 3.3 grams

(11) LIME PINEAPPLE CREAMY JELLO - 6 Servings

1 cup plain yogu

165

Low Carb & No Carb Cookbook. (A) 130-Recipes. (B) 85-Low Carb Desserts. (C) 27-Restaurant Guide To Eating Out.

rt (11.2 grams) 1 box sugar free lime jello
1/2 cup pineapple chunks (10 grams)

Prepare jello according to package directions. mix in yogurt and pineapple. Pour into 6 small bowls and chill. For variety, use kiwi jello & 1 cup sliced kiwi.

Carb Count: Recipe Total 21.2 grams, Per Serving 3.5 grams

(12) <u>LEMON CREPES - 3 Servings</u>

1 egg
4 egg whites
1/4 cup high gluten flour (7.5 grams) 1/4 cup Splenda (6 grams)
1 tbsp light cream (0.3 grams) 1 1/2 tsp vanilla extract

166
Low Carb & No Carb Cookbook. (A) 130-Recipes. (B) 85-Low Carb Desserts. (C) 27-Restaurant Guide To Eating Out.

2 tsp grated lemon zest (0.6 grams)
3/4 cup cottage cheese (4.5 grams)

In a medium bowl, combine the egg, egg whites, flour, Splenda, cream, vanilla and lemon zest and stir to combine. Add cottage cheese to the flour mixture and stir to blend. Heat a large nonstick skillet over medium heat. Spoon the batter by spoonfuls into the hot skillet and when holes appear in the pancakes, turn and cook for 1 to 2 minutes longer, until golden. Repeat until all the batter is used. Serve with strawberries and cream cheese (or sour cream or creme fraiche or cottage cheese).

Carb Count: Recipe Total 18.9 grams, Per Serving 6.3 grams

(13) CHOCOLATE CREPES - 4 Servings

1 egg
4 egg whites
1/4 cup high gluten flour (7.5 grams)
1/4 cup Splenda (6 grams)
2 tbsp light cream (0.6 grams)
2 tbsp cocoa powder (2.5 grams)
3/4 cup cottage cheese (4.5 grams)

In a medium bowl, combine the egg, egg whites, flour, Splenda, cream and cocoa

167

Low Carb & No Carb Cookbook. (A) 130-Recipes. (B) 85-Low Carb Desserts. (C) 27-Restaurant Guide To Eating Out.

powder. Stir to combine. Add cottage cheese and stir to blend. Heat a large nonstick skillet over medium heat. Spoon the batter by spoonfuls into the hot skillet and cook until all the batter is used. Serve with strawberries and cream cheese (or sour cream or creme fraiche or cottage cheese).

Carb Count: Recipe Total 21.1 grams, Per Serving 5.3 grams

(14) BUTTERSCOTCH PUDDING - 3 Servings

1 cup cream (9.6 grams)
3/4 cup water 1 package sugar-free butterscotch pudding (8 grams) whipped cream (3.3 grams per prepared cup)

Combine cream, water and pudding mix and blend on high for 15 seconds. Immediately pour into 8 single serve dishes. Chill for 5 minutes or overnight. Top with whipped cream.

Carb Count: Recipe Total 17.6 grams, Per Serving 5.7 grams

(15) COCONUT CHOCOLATE PUDDING - 4 Servings

1 cup cream (9.6 grams)
1 cup water
1 package. sugar-free chocolate pudding (8

grams) 1/2 cup
unsweetened, shredded
coconut (6.1 grams)
whipped cream (3.3 grams per prepared cup)

Place cream and water in blender. Add pudding &
coconut and blend on high for 15 seconds. Immediately pour into 8 single serve dishes. Chill for 5 minutes or overnight. Top with whipped cream.

Carb Count: Recipe Total 23.7 grams, Per Serving 5.9 grams

16. TAPIOCA PUDDING - 8 servings
1 cup Splenda (24 grams)
6 scoops vanilla protein powder, optional
6 tbsp tapioca (20 grams)
3 cup cream (28.7 grams)
2 cup water
1 egg

Combine ingredients. Let stand for five minutes. In saucepan, place over a medium heat. Heat, stirring until mixture comes to a full boil. Remove from heat. Stir in two teaspoons vanilla and allow to stand for 20 minutes. Serve warm or chilled.

Carb Count: Recipe Total 48.8 grams, Per Serving 9.1 grams

(17) CHEWY COCONUT BARS - 4 Servings

169
Low Carb & No Carb Cookbook. (A) 130-Recipes. (B) 85-Low Carb Desserts. (C) 27-Restaurant Guide To Eating Out.

4 egg whites
1 cup Splenda (24 grams)
1/4 teaspoon maple flavoring
1/4 cup butter, melted
1 tsp vanilla (1.5 grams)
1/2 cup high gluten flour (12 grams)
1 tsp baking powder
1/4 tsp salt
3/4 cup unsweetened coconut, finely chopped (9.1 grams)

Beat eggs, sweetener and maple flavoring in medium bowl; mix in margarine and vanilla. Combine flour, baking powder and salt in small bowl; stir into egg mixture. Mix in coconut and raisins. Spread batter evenly in greased 8-inch square baking pan. Bake in preheated 350"F oven until browned and toothpick inserted in center comes out clean, about 20 minutes. Cool in pan on wire rack; cut into squares. Carb Count: Recipe Total 46.1 grams, Per Serving 11.5 grams

(18) RASPBERRY BRULEE - 8 Servings

170

Low Carb & No Carb Cookbook. (A) 130-Recipes. (B) 85-Low Carb Desserts. (C) 27-Restaurant Guide To Eating Out.

2 cup heavy cream (19.8 grams)
1 tbsp cornstarch
1/2 cup Splenda (12 grams)
2 egg whites, lightly beaten
1 tsp vanilla
4 ounces cream cheese (8 grams)
1/2 cup fresh raspberries (7.1 grams)

Combine cream & cornstarch in double boiler until completely dissolved. Add Splenda & egg whites. Mix well. Place double boiler over simmering water & cook, stirring constantly, until thickens. Remove from heat and stir in vanilla. Add cream cheese & stir until mixture is smooth. Fold in raspberries & divide among 8 ramekins. Cover & chill for 2 hours.
Broil until top browns. Serve.

Carb Count: Recipe Total 46.9 grams, Per Serving 5.8 grams

(19) PEACHES & RICOTTA - 4 Servings

2 ripe peaches,
quartered, pits removed
(8 grams) 1/8 cup
Splenda (3 grams)

1/3 cup whole milk ricotta cheese (0.6 grams)
1/2 cup cottage cheese (3 grams)

Mix ricotta, cottage cheese & Splenda. Spoon mixture into middle of each peach. Preheat broiler. Cook under a broiler for 5-9 minutes or until peaches are hot.

171

Low Carb & No Carb Cookbook. (A) 130-Recipes. (B) 85-Low Carb Desserts. (C) 27-Restaurant Guide To Eating Out.

Carb Count: Recipe Total 14.6 grams, Per Serving 3.6 grams

(20) <u>PEACH SOUFFLE - 4 Servings</u>

2 peaches (18 grams)
1/2 cup Splenda (12 grams)
1/2 tsp lemon juice (0.2 grams)
1/4 tsp salt
4 egg whites

Heat oven to 350 degrees. Spray 4 individual souffle dishes (1 cup capacity). Peel peach and cut into thin slices. Sprinkle with 1 tablespoon of sugar and the lemon juice. Beat egg whites with salt until they hold soft peaks. Gradually beat in the remaining sugar and continue beating until the whites hold stiff peaks. Gently fold in peach slices. Divide among dishes and smooth tops. Bake until puffed and browned, about 18 minutes. Serve immediately.

Carb Count: Recipe Total 30.2 grams, Per Serving 7.5 grams

(21) <u>BROWNIE TORTE - 5 Servings</u>

1/2 cup high gluten flour (12 grams)
1 tbsp cocoa (2.7 grams)
1/2 tsp cinnamon (1 grams)
1 tbsp espresso or coffee (liquid)
2 ounces bitter chocolate (8 grams)1/2 cup
   cream cheese (4 grams)

Low Carb & No Carb Cookbook. (A) 130-Recipes. (B) 85-Low Carb Desserts. (C) 27-Restaurant Guide To Eating Out.

1 cup Splenda (24 grams)
1 tsp vanilla (1.5 grams)
2 eggs

Preheat oven to 325 degrees. For filling, combine flour with cocoa & cinnamon. Melt chocolate over double boiler & combine with espresso. Blend cream cheese, sugar, vanilla & eggs. Add chocolate mix to cream cheese mix. Gradually stir in flour mix. Pour into prepared crust.
Bake for 30 minutes.

Carb Count: Recipe Total 53.2 grams, Per Serving 10.6 grams

(22) CREAMY CAPPUCCINO - 2 Servings

2 tbsp cold water
1 envelope unflavored gelatin
1/4 cup boiling water
3 tbsp instant cappuccino powder
2 tbsp Splenda (3 grams)
1 cup cream (9.4 grams)

173
Low Carb & No Carb Cookbook. (A) 130-Recipes. (B) 85-Low Carb Desserts. (C) 27-Restaurant Guide To Eating Out.

Place cold water in a bowl & sprinkle with gelatin. Let stand for 5 minutes. Add boiling water & stir until gelatin is dissolved. Add cappuccino powder & Splenda. Stir until dissolved. Add cream & mix well. Cover & refrigerate for 3 hours.

Carb Count: Recipe Total 12.4 grams, Per Serving 6.2 grams

(23) VANILLA CUSTARD - 4 Servings

1 1/2 cup cream (13.8 grams)
1/2 cup water
1/4 cup Splend

Low Carb & No Carb Cookbook. (A) 130-Recipes. (B) 85-Low Carb Desserts. (C) 27-Restaurant Guide To Eating Out.

a (6 grams)

5 egg yolks

1 tsp vanilla (1.5 grams)

Warm cream and water over low heat. Beat Splenda with egg yolks. Slowly add cream to eggs, beating constantly. Blend in vanilla and pour into custard cups. Place in a pan of hot water and bake at 325 degrees F for 1 hour. Chill and serve.

Carb Count: Recipe Total 21.3 grams, Per Serving 5.3 grams

175
Low Carb & No Carb Cookbook. (A) 130-Recipes. (B) 85-Low Carb Desserts. (C) 27-Restaurant Guide To Eating Out.

(24) CHOCOLATE CHEESECAKE - 8 Servings

32 oz cottage cheese (24 grams)
3 packets unflavored gelatin
3/4 cup warm water
1 1/2 cup Splenda (36 grams)
1 cup sour cream (16

176

Low Carb & No Carb Cookbook. (A) 130-Recipes. (B) 85-Low Carb Desserts. (C) 27-Restaurant Guide To Eating Out.

grams)
3 tbsp cocoa (3.9 grams)

Dissolve gelatin in water. Blend with cottage cheese, sour cream, sweetener & cocoa until smooth. Line pie pan with chocolate wafers. Pour cottage cheese mix over crust. Refrigerate overnight.

Carb Count: Recipe Total 79.9 grams, Per Serving 9.9 grams

(25) <u>STRAWBERRY CHEESECAKE - 6 Servings</u>

1 cup crushed pecans (15 grams) mixed with 1 tbsp melted butter
1/2 cup Splenda (12 grams)
1 package (8 ounces) cream cheese, softened (16 grams)
1 tsp vanilla (1.5 grams)
1 tbsp Splenda
1 cup cold water
2 tbsp cornstarch
1 package sugar-free strawberry gelatin 1 pint strawberries (10.4 grams), hulled, sliced
whipped cream (3.3 grams per cup)

Beat cream cheese, vanilla, and Splenda in small bowl until fluffy; spread evenly in bottom of pie pan. Mix cold water and

177

Low Carb & No Carb Cookbook. (A) 130-Recipes. (B) 85-Low Carb Desserts. (C) 27-Restaurant Guide To Eating Out.

cornstarch in small saucepan; heat to boiling, whisking constantly until thickened, about 1 minute. Add gelatin and sweetener, whisking until gelatin is dissolved. Cool 10 minutes. Arrange half of the strawberries over the cream cheese; spoon half the gelatin mixture over strawberries. Arrange remaining strawberries over pie and spoon on remaining gelatin mixture. Refrigerate until pie is set and chilled, 1 to 2 hours. Serve with whipped topping, if desired.

Carb Count: Recipe Total 44.5 grams, Per Serving 7.4 grams

(26) LEMON SHERBET -
6 Servings

juice and zest of 2 lemons (6 grams)
2 egg yolks
3 cup light cream (13.5 grams)
1/2 cup liquid sweetener

Blend all ingredients well. Pour into ice cream maker and follow manufacturer's instructions.

Carb Count: Recipe Total 19.5 grams, Per Serving 3.2 grams

(27) WALNUT TORTE - 6 Servings

178
Low Carb & No Carb Cookbook. (A) 130-Recipes. (B) 85-Low Carb Desserts. (C) 27-Restaurant Guide To Eating Out.

3/4 cup ground walnuts - especially good with crispy nuts RECIPE# 83 (9 grams)
1 1/4 cups Splenda (18 grams)
4 egg whites, r

179
Low Carb & No Carb Cookbook. (A) 130-Recipes. (B) 85-Low Carb Desserts. (C) 27-Restaurant Guide To Eating Out.

oom tempt sp vanilla (1.5 grams)
1 1/2 cup cream (13.8 grams)
2 tsp lemon zest (0.4 grams)

Beat egg whites until glossy. Gradually add 1/2 cup Splenda, beating until stiff. Beat in 1/2 tsp vanilla. Fold over two pie plates lined with ground walnuts. Bake at 300 degrees F for 1 1/2 hours. Turn oven off and leave in the oven for another hour. Beat whipping cream with 1/2 cup Splenda,

180

Low Carb & No Carb Cookbook. (A) 130-Recipes. (B) 85-Low Carb Desserts. (C) 27-Restaurant Guide To Eating Out.

lemon zest and 1/2 tsp vanilla until stiff. Layer walnut meringue and icing.

Carb Count: Recipe Total 33.7 grams, Per Serving 5.6 grams

(28) **STRAWBERRIES & CREAM COOKIES - 6 Servings**

8 ounces cream cheese (16 grams)
3 cold egg whites1/2 cup Splenda (12 grams)
1/4 cup high gluten flour (6 grams)
2 tsp strawberry extract

Preheat oven to 350 degrees. Beat egg whites in a glass or metal bowl until foamy. Add remaining ingredients and mix well. Drop teaspoon of batter on greased cookie sheet. Bake for 15 minutes or until lightly browned. Serve with strawberries (10.4 grams).

Carb Count: Recipe Total 34 grams, Per Serving 5.6 grams

(29) **PEANUT BUTTER CHOCOLATE CUPS - 4 Servings**

2 tbsp butter
1/3 cup peanut butter (12 grams; check your brand)
1 oz unsweetened chocolate (4 grams)
1/3 cup cottage cheese (2 grams)

181
Low Carb & No Carb Cookbook. (A) 130-Recipes. (B) 85-Low Carb Desserts. (C) 27-Restaurant Guide To Eating Out.

1/2 cup Splenda (12 grams)

Melt butter, peanut butter and chocolate in microwave. Cool slightly, then add cottage cheese, sweetener and vanilla. Spoon onto wax paper and refrigerate.

Carb Count: Recipe Total 30 grams, Per Serving 7.5 grams

(30) RASPBERRY MERINGUES - 6 Servings

3 egg whites
1/2 cup Splenda (12 grams)
4 ounces cream cheese (8 grams) 1/2 cup ricotta cheese (0.9 grams)
1/2 cup raspberries (7.1 grams)

Preheat oven to 275 degrees F. Whisk egg whites until stiff, gradually add 1/4 cup Splenda. Spoon mixture onto two greased baking sheet, spreading meringue into two 8 inch circles. Bake for 1 1/2 - 2 hours or until crisp and dry. Mix cream cheese with 1/4 cup Splenda and ricotta cheese and raspberries. Place one meringue on decorative plate. Layer with cream cheese and top with second meringue.

Carb Count: Recipe Total 28 grams, Per Serving 4.6 grams

(31) BREAD PUDDING - 2 Servings

3 oz bag plain pork rinds, lightly crushed

182

Low Carb & No Carb Cookbook. (A) 130-Recipes. (B) 85-Low Carb Desserts. (C) 27-Restaurant Guide To Eating Out.

2 eggs
1/2 cup cream (4.7 grams)
1/2 cup water
1/2 cups Splenda

183
Low Carb & No Carb Cookbook. (A) 130-Recipes. (B) 85-Low Carb Desserts. (C) 27-Restaurant Guide To Eating Out.

(12 grams) 1 tsp vanilla (0.7 grams)
1 tsp cinnamon (1.8 grams)

Mix cream, eggs, water, sweetener, vanilla and cinnamon. Butter glass dish. Put lightly crushed pork rinds in dish and pour cream mixture into dish. Preheat oven to 350 and let casserole sit while it preheats so pork rinds can absorb some liquid. Sprinkle with cinnamon. Bake 30-

184

Low Carb & No Carb Cookbook. (A) 130-Recipes. (B) 85-Low Carb Desserts. (C) 27-Restaurant Guide To Eating Out.

40 minutes until top lightly browned. Serve warm.

Carb Count: Recipe Total 19.2 grams, Per Serving 9.6 grams

(32) <u>CHOCOLATE PEANUT BUTTER PARFAITS - 6 Servings</u>

1 1/2 cup cream (13.6 grams)
2 tbsp chunky peanut butter (6 grams; check your brand)
1 package sugar free chocolate pudding mix (8 grams)

Whip cream.. Fold in peanut butter. Prepare pudding according to package directions. Fill parfait glasses with alternating layers of peanut butter whipped cream and pudding. Chill and serve.

Carb Count: Recipe Total 27.6 grams, Per Serving 4.5 grams

(33) <u>CHOCOLATE FROSTY - 4 Servings</u>

1 cup heavy cream (6.6 grams)
1 tsp vanilla extract (1.5 grams)
2 packages sugar free cocoa mix (8 grams)

Beat cream and add vanilla. When soft peaks form, gradually add cocoa mix. Continue beating until stiff peaks form (about 30 seconds). Freeze for 30 minutes. Stir. Freeze for 20 minutes. Stir. Freeze for 15 minutes. Enjoy!

185

Low Carb & No Carb Cookbook. (A) 130-Recipes. (B) 85-Low Carb Desserts. (C) 27-Restaurant Guide To Eating Out.

Carb Count: Recipe Total 16.1 grams, Per Serving 4 grams

(34) <u>CHOCOLATE PEANUT BUTTER PIE - 12 Servings</u>

1 cup crushed or ground pecans (15 grams)
1 tbsp melted butter
2 tbsp butter
1 oz unsweetened chocolate (4 grams)
2 tbsp light cream (0.5 grams) 1 tsp vanilla (1.5 grams)
1 cup Splenda (24 grams)
1/8 cup peanut butter (6 grams; check your brand)
4 oz cream cheese (4 grams)

Mix pecans and butter. Pour in pie plate, spread to cover bottom of plate and place in freezer.
Then, mix melted butter and chocolate in small saucepan. Heat & stir. Mix in cream and vanilla. Add Splenda. Pour over frozen pie crust and place in freezer again. Next, mix peanut butter and cream cheese. Blend well. Spread over frozen pie. Serve with whipped topping.

Carb Count: Recipe Total 55 grams, Per Serving 4.5 grams

186

Low Carb & No Carb Cookbook. (A) 130-Recipes. (B) 85-Low Carb Desserts. (C) 27-Restaurant Guide To Eating Out.

(35) <u>PEANUT BUTTER COOKIES - 12 Servings</u>

2 eggs
1/2 cup Splenda (12 grams)
1/2 cup butter
1/2 cup peanut butter (24 grams; check your brand)
1 tsp vanilla (1.5 grams)
1/8 tsp salt
1/4 tsp baking soda
1/2 cup milk & egg protein powder

In mixing bowl, cream butter and Splenda. Add eggs and beat well. Add peanut butter and vanilla and blend well. Add protein powder, salt and
baking soda. Mix to form a moderately stiff dough. Place by rounded teaspoons on cookie sheet, press down with fork, and bake in preheated 300 oven for 15-20 minutes.

Carb Count: Recipe Total 37.5 grams, Per Serving 3.1 grams

(36) <u>ZUCCHINI APPLES - 4 Servings</u>

3 small zucchini, peeled and sliced (10 grams)
1/4 tsp cinnamon (0.4 grams)
pinch of nutmeg
1/4 cup Splenda (6 grams)
2 tbsp melted butter

Combine all ingredients in glass dish & bake for 350 degrees for 30 minutes.

187

Low Carb & No Carb Cookbook. (A) 130-Recipes. (B) 85-Low Carb Desserts. (C) 27-Restaurant Guide To Eating Out.

Carb Count: Recipe Total 16.4 grams, Per Serving 4.1 grams

(37) <u>CHOCOLATE CHEESE CAKE MUFFINS - 6 Servings</u>

8 oz softened cream cheese (8 grams)
1 egg
1 tsp vanilla extract (1.5 grams)
1 package chocolate pudding mix (8 grams)

Mix together with mixer until creamy. Fill 6 greased muffin tins. Bake at 350 degrees F for 20 minutes.

Carb Count: Recipe Total 17.5 grams, Per Serving 2.9 grams

(38) <u>CHOCOLATE SHAKE - 2 Servings</u>

1/4 cup light cream (1.5 grams)
1/4 cup cottage cheese (1.5 grams) 1/22 cup water
1 tbsp cocoa (2.7 grams)
1/4 cup Splenda (6 grams)
Ice

Combine ingredients in blender & enjoy!

Carb Count: Recipe Total 11.7 grams, Per Serving 5.8 grams

(39) <u>COFFEE & CREAM ICEE - 4 Servings</u>

188

Low Carb & No Carb Cookbook. (A) 130-Recipes. (B) 85-Low Carb Desserts. (C) 27-Restaurant Guide To Eating Out.

cup espresso 2 cup cream (18.2 grams)

189
Low Carb & No Carb Cookbook. (A) 130-Recipes. (B) 85-Low Carb Desserts. (C) 27-Restaurant Guide To Eating Out.

liquid sweetener to taste

1 cup crushed ice

Combine in blender & enjoy!

Carb Count: Recipe Total 18.2 grams, Per Serving 4.5 grams

(40) <u>SUGAR COOKIES - 12 Servings</u>

1 cup almond flour (48 grams)

190
Low Carb & No Carb Cookbook. (A) 130-Recipes. (B) 85-Low Carb Desserts. (C) 27-Restaurant Guide To Eating Out.

1 cup Splenda (24 grams)

1 egg

1/2 cup softened butter

Preheat oven to 350 Degrees F. Mix almond flour and Splenda.. In aseparate bowl, lightly beat egg and then mix well with butter. Add to dry ingredients and mix. Form small balls and place on two cookie sheets. Bake for 7-9 minutes. Makes 2 dozen cookies.

191
Low Carb & No Carb Cookbook. (A) 130-Recipes. (B) 85-Low Carb Desserts. (C) 27-Restaurant Guide To Eating Out.

Carb Count: Recipe Total 72 grams, Per Serving 6 grams

(41) <u>STRAWBERRY ICE CREAM - 12 Servings</u>

2 cup strawberries (20 grams)
3 cup light cream (28.9 grams)
2/3 cup Splenda (16 grams)
1 tsp vanilla extract

Put blended strawberries in ice cream maker container, add remaining ingredients. Mix with spoon until well blended. Follow machines instructions for freezing.

Carb Count: Recipe Total 64.9 grams, Per Serving 5.4 grams

(42) <u>CHOCOLATE CAKE - 6 Servings</u>

6 tbsp butter
4 ounces unsweetened chocolate (16 grams)
1/3 cup light cream (1.5 grams)
1/3 cup strawberry all fruit jam (13 grams; check your brand)
1 tsp espresso powder
2 tbsp Splenda (3 grams)
3 large eggs
1 tsp vanilla
1
c
u
p
S

192
Low Carb & No Carb Cookbook. (A) 130-Recipes. (B) 85-Low Carb Desserts. (C) 27-Restaurant Guide To Eating Out.

pl en da (24 grams) 1/8 tsp cream of tartar
1/4 cup flour (6 grams)
1/8 tsp salt

Preheat oven to 350 degrees F. Grease cake pan & dust with cocoa powder.

193
Low Carb & No Carb Cookbook. (A) 130-Recipes. (B) 85-Low Carb Desserts. (C) 27-Restaurant Guide To Eating Out.

Set aside. Combine butter, chocolate, cream, jam, and espresso powder. Melt in a double boiler on low heat (or in microwave, 2-3 minutes in a microwave-safe dish). Let cool. Separate eggs. Combine flour & salt. Set aside. Add sugar, egg yolks, and vanilla to chocolate mix. Add sweetener & blend until smooth. In another bowl, beat egg whites until foamy. Add cream of tartar and beta into stiff peaks. Fold in cooled chocolate mix. Pour into prepared pan. Bake 18-20 minutes or until toothpick comes out clean. Cool. Refrigerate 1-2 hours. Serve with whipped cream & strawberries (5.2 grams per half cup) (or Chocolate Frosting, RECIPE #63).

Carb Count: Recipe Total 63.5 grams, Per Serving 10.5 grams

(43) CHOCOLATE FROSTING - 6 Servings

1/4 cup sugar free chocolate pudding mix (8 grams)
1 cup cream (9.3 grams)
1
/
4

c
u
p

S
p
l
e
n

194
Low Carb & No Carb Cookbook. (A) 130-Recipes. (B) 85-Low Carb Desserts. (C) 27-Restaurant Guide To Eating Out.

da (6 grams) 1 tsp of vanilla (1.5 gr

195
Low Carb & No Carb Cookbook. (A) 130-Recipes. (B) 85-Low Carb Desserts. (C) 27-Restaurant Guide To Eating Out.

ams)

4 oz cream cheese, softened (4 grams)

Mix well. Thin with cream or water as needed.

Carb Count: Recipe Total 28.8 grams, Per Serving 4.8 grams

(44) CINNAMON PECAN MUFFINS - 6 Servings

1/3 cup pecans (5 grams) chopped finely
1/2 tsp. cinnamon (0.4 grams)
1/2 cup Splenda (12 grams)
3 large eggs separated and at room temperature
3/4 cup protein powder
3/4 tsp baking powder
1/4 tsp salt
1/4 tsp cream of tartar
3 tbsp sour cream (3

196
Low Carb & No Carb Cookbook. (A) 130-Recipes. (B) 85-Low Carb Desserts. (C) 27-Restaurant Guide To Eating Out.

grams)
1 tbsp butter
1/2 tsp vanilla (0.7 grams)
2 tsp almond extract

Combine pecans, cinnamon, and 1/4 cup Splenda and mix well. Set aside for toppings. Preheat oven to 325 degrees F. Beat egg whites with cream of tartar until stiff but not dry. Separately, beat egg yolks. Add sour cream, extracts, and remaining sweetener and beat thoroughly. Combine protein powder, baking powder, and salt and mix into the yolk mixture. Stir until combined, and then gently fold in the egg whites. Fill greased muffin tins halfway. Top with nut mixture and bake in preheated oven for 50-60 minutes.

Carb Count: Recipe Total 21.1 grams, Per Serving 3.5 grams

(45) CINNAMON ROLLS - 4 Servings

4 eggs
2 tbsp cottage cheese (0.8 grams)

197

Low Carb & No Carb Cookbook. (A) 130-Recipes. (B) 85-Low Carb Desserts. (C) 27-Restaurant Guide To Eating Out.

1/4 cup Splenda (6 grams)

1 stick but

198

Low Carb & No Carb Cookbook. (A) 130-Recipes. (B) 85-Low Carb Desserts. (C) 27-Restaurant Guide To Eating Out.

t
e
r

1/2 tsp cinnamon (0.4 grams)

Separate the 4 eggs. Whip whites with a pinch of salt until stiff peaks form. In a food processor, blend egg yolks, 2 tbsp, cottage cheese and Splenda. Gently fold yolks into whites. Spread into 6 mounds on greased cookie sheet. Bake at 300 for 30-40 minutes. Combine butter with cinnamon & 2 tbsp Splenda. Serve with rolls.

Carb Count: Recipe Total 7.2 grams, Per Serving 1.8 grams

(46) <u>LOW CARB POPOVERS- 6 Servings</u>

1/2 cup gluten flour (12 grams)
1/2
cup
regul
ar
flour
(12
gram
s) 2
eggs
1/2 cup heavy cream (4.8 grams)
3/4 cup water
1/2 tsp salt
1 tbsp melted butter

199
Low Carb & No Carb Cookbook. (A) 130-Recipes. (B) 85-Low Carb Desserts. (C) 27-Restaurant Guide To Eating Out.

Preheat oven to 450 degrees. Combine all ingredients and pour into generously buttered muffin tins.
Bake for 20 minutes at 450 degrees, then turn down oven to 350 degrees and bake 10-15 minutes until golden browned.

Carb Count: Recipe Total 28.8 grams, Per Serving 4.8 grams

(47) VANILLA ICE CREAM - 12 Servings

10 egg yolks
2 1/2 quarts heavy cream (25 grams)
1 whole vanilla bean
2 tsp vanilla extract (3 grams)
1/2 cup Splenda, or to taste (12 grams)

Beat egg yolks 3- 5 minutes. In large saucepan simmer cream with vanilla bean for 30 minutes. Discard vanilla bean. Temper by pouring some of cream mixture into eggs slowly. Slowly mix all eggs into pan mixture. Simmer until thick. Add sweeteners and vanilla extract. Strain into chilled bowl. Freeze in ice cream maker.

Carb Count: Recipe Total 40 grams, Per Serving 3.1 grams

(48) CHEESECAKE - 12 Servings

200

Low Carb & No Carb Cookbook. (A) 130-Recipes. (B) 85-Low Carb Desserts. (C) 27-Restaurant Guide To Eating Out.

2 cup sour cream (32 grams)
1 tsp vanilla (1.5 grams)
1 tbsp Splenda (1.5 grams)
24 ounces cream cheese, softened (54 grams)
1 cup Splenda

201
Low Carb & No Carb Cookbook. (A) 130-Recipes. (B) 85-Low Carb Desserts. (C) 27-Restaurant Guide To Eating Out.

(24 grams)

4 eggs

1 tsp vanilla (1.5 grams)

In a bowl, mix the sour cream, vanilla and 1 tbsp Splenda until well combined. Cover with plastic wrap and refrigerate. In a large bowl, beat the cream cheese and 1 cup Splenda until fluffy. Add the eggs, one at a time, blending well after each addition. Blend in the remaining 1 teaspoon vanilla. Pour the cream cheese mixture into the greased pie pan and bake at 350 degree for 50 minutes. Spread the sour cream mixture over the top and bake an additional 5 minutes. Chill and Serve.

Carb Count: Recipe Total 122.5 grams, Per Serving 10.2 grams

(49) **LEMON ALMOND CAKE - 4 Servings**

1 cup blanched slivered almonds (20 grams)
1/2 cup Splenda (12 grams)
4 eggs, separated
5 tsp grated lemon peel (1.2 grams)
1/2 tsp cinnamon (0.9 grams)
Pinch of salt

Preheat oven to 375EF. Butter cake pan. Line bottom of pan with waxed paper. Finely grind almonds with 2 tablespoons Splenda in processor. Combine yolks, 2 tablespoons Splenda, lemon peel, cinnamon and salt in medium bowl. Using electric mixer, beat until thick and smooth, about 2 minutes. Stir in almond mixture. Using clean beaters, beat egg whites in large bowl until soft peaks form. Gradually add 4 tablespoons Splenda, beating until stiff but not dry. Fold large spoonful of whites into almond mixture. Gently fold in remaining whites. Transfer batter to pan. Bake until toothpick comes out clean, about 35 minutes. Cool in pan on rack. Turn out onto platter.

Carb Count: Recipe Total 34.1 grams, Per Serving 8.5 grams

(50) FRENCH SILK PIE - 4 Servings

1/2 cup butter
3/4 cup Splenda (18 grams)
2 oz unsweetened baking chocolate (8 grams)
1 tsp vanilla (3 grams)
2 eggs

203

Low Carb & No Carb Cookbook. (A) 130-Recipes. (B) 85-Low Carb Desserts. (C) 27-Restaurant Guide To Eating Out.

Cream butter and Splenda. Melt chocolate and blend into butter/sweetener mixture when cooled. Stir in vanilla. Add eggs, one at a time. Beat well. Chill 1-2 hours minimum. Top with whipped cream (3.3 grams per cup) if desired.

Carb Count: Recipe Total 29 grams, Per Serving 7.25 grams

(51) <u>CREME BRULEE - 6 Servings</u>

1 ¼ quarts of heavy cream (12.5 grams)
1 tsp vanilla.
1 cup Splenda (24 grams)
12 egg yolks

Combine heavy cream, vanilla and 1/2 cup Splenda to a boil. Combine the beaten egg yolks and remaining 1/2 cup Splenda. Combine cream with yolk mixture. Fill ramekins, place in water bath
Bake in a 325 F (165 CUP) oven until just barely set, approximately 45 minutes. Remove from water bath when cool, wipe bottoms of ramekins, and refrigerate overnight.

Carb Count: Recipe Total 36.5 grams, Per Serving 6 grams

(52) <u>ORANGE CHOCOLATE CREAM - 6 Servings</u>

2 oz unsweetened chocolate (8 grams)
1 tbsp butter

204

Low Carb & No Carb Cookbook. (A) 130-Recipes. (B) 85-Low Carb Desserts. (C) 27-Restaurant Guide To Eating Out.

2 packages unflavored gelatin 2 ice cubes
1 tsp grated orange peel
2 cup whipping cream (19.2 grams)
3/4 cup Splenda (18 grams)
1/8 cup unsweetened cocoa powder (5.5 grams)

Melt chocolate with butter. Place the gelatin in a small bowl. Add 1 cup boiling water and orange peel. Stir until gelatin in dissolved. Add ice. Beat whipping cream. Add Splenda and cocoa powder. Slowly add in chocolate mixture. Then add gelatin mixture. Beat well. Chill for at least 3 hours.

Carb Count: Recipe Total 50.7 grams, Per Serving 8.4 grams

(53) COCONUT CREME PIE - 6 Servings

4 eggs
1/4 cup butter
1 cup Splenda (24 grams) 1/4 tsp salt
1/2 tsp baking powder
2 cup heavy whipping cream (19.2 grams)
1 cup unsweetened coconut (12.2 grams)
1 tsp vanilla extract (1.5 grams)

Place all ingredients in blender at one time and blend until mixed together. Pour into a buttered 10-inch pie dish. Bake in a 350 degree oven for 1 hour.

205
Low Carb & No Carb Cookbook. (A) 130-Recipes. (B) 85-Low Carb Desserts. (C) 27-Restaurant Guide To Eating Out.

Carb Count: Recipe Total 56.9 grams, Per Serving 9.4 grams

(54) **TIRAMISU - 4 Servings**

1 container marscapone cheese
1/2 cups Splenda (12 grams)
2 tbsp coff

206
Low Carb & No Carb Cookbook. (A) 130-Recipes. (B) 85-Low Carb Desserts. (C) 27-Restaurant Guide To Eating Out.

e
e
4 tsp cocoa powder (4 grams)

Beat the marscapone until it is creamy. Add 2 tablespoons coffee and blend. Add Splenda. Chill & serve with cocoa powder sprinkled on top.

Carb Count: Recipe Total 16 grams, Per Serving 4 grams

(55) <u>PEACHES AND CREAM- 6 Servings</u>

1 cup ricotta cheese (7.5 grams)
1/2 cup cream (4.8 grams)
1 cup peaches, chopped (18.8 grams)
1 tsp almond extract
1/4 cup Splenda (6 grams)

Combine ingredients. Chill & enjoy!

Carb Count: Recipe Total 37.1 grams, Per Serving 6 grams

(56) <u>RASPBERRY ICE CREAM - 10 Servings</u>

207

Low Carb & No Carb Cookbook. (A) 130-Recipes. (B) 85-Low Carb Desserts. (C) 27-Restaurant Guide To Eating Out.

1 cup raspberries (14.2 grams) 1 1/2 cup Splenda (36 grams)
2 tbsp lemon juice (2.6 grams)
4 cup heavy cream (38.2 grams)
1 tsp vanilla extract (1.5 grams)

In a 3-quart saucepan combine raspberries, Splenda and lemon juice. Mash berries slightly and cook over medium heat, stirring occasionally, until the mixture comes to a boil. Simmer 5 minutes.
Remove from heat and puree in a blender. Cool the mixture. Add cream and vanilla. Freeze according to manufacturer's directions.

Carb Count: Recipe Total 92.5 grams, Per Serving 9.25 grams

(57) **PECAN ICE CREAM - 10 Servings**

4 cup heavy cream (38.2 grams)
1

c
u
p

S
p
l
e
n
d
a

208
Low Carb & No Carb Cookbook. (A) 130-Recipes. (B) 85-Low Carb Desserts. (C) 27-Restaurant Guide To Eating Out.

(24 grams)

2 tbsp butter

1 tsp vanilla extract (1.5 grams)
1/2 cup toasted pecans (10 grams)

Combine the half of the cream, Splenda, and butter in a medium saucepan. Cook, stirring constantly over low heat until bubbles form around the edges of the pan. Let the mixture cool and put it in the ice cream machine. Stir in the rest of the cream and vanilla. Freeze as directed by your machine's manufacturer. Add pecans after ice cream begins toharden.

209
Low Carb & No Carb Cookbook. (A) 130-Recipes. (B) 85-Low Carb Desserts. (C) 27-Restaurant Guide To Eating Out.

Carb Count: Recipe Total 73.7 grams, Per Serving 7.3 grams

(58) <u>CHOCOLATE ICE CREAM - 10 Servings</u>

2 oz unsweetened chocolate (8 grams)
1/4 cup unsweetened cocoa powder (11 grams)
2 eggs
1 cup Splenda (24 grams)
2 cup whipping cream (19.2 grams) 1/2 cup water
1 tsp vanilla extract (1.5 grams)

Melt the unsweetened chocolate on top of a double boiler over hot water. Gradually whisk in the cocoa and heat, stirring constantly, until smooth. Whisk in the cream and water. Combine well & remove from heat. In a bowl, whisk the eggs until light and fluffy, 1 to 2 minutes. Whisk in the Splenda until blended, about 1 minute more. Pour into the cream and vanilla and whisk to blend. Pour the chocolate mixture into the cream mixture and blend. Cover and refrigerate until cold. Transfer the mixture to an ice cream maker and freeze following the manufacturer's instructions.

Carb Count: Recipe Total 63.7 grams, Per Serving 6.3 grams

(59) <u>PEANUT BUTTER ICE CREAM - 10 Servings</u>

210
Low Carb & No Carb Cookbook. (A) 130-Recipes. (B) 85-Low Carb Desserts. (C) 27-Restaurant Guide To Eating Out.

2 eggs
1/2 cup Splenda (12 grams)
1/2 cup sugar free chunky peanut butter (24 grams; check your brand)
3 cup heavy cream (28.8 grams)

Whisk together the eggs and sugar until light and fluffy. Add the peanut butter and whisk until smooth. Mix in the whipping cream. Transfer the mixture to the ice cream maker and process according to manufacturer's instructions.

Carb Count: Recipe Total 64.8 grams, Per Serving 6.4 grams

(60) COFFEE ICE CREAM - 4 Servings

6 egg yolks
1/2 cup Splenda (12 grams)
2 cup cream (19.2 grams)
4 cup coffee

Beat the egg yolks with the Splenda. Add cream & coffee. Put in pan & heat until the sauce thickens and coats the back of the spoon. Freeze according to manufacturer's instructions.
Carb Count: Recipe Total 31.2 grams, Per Serving 7.8 grams

(61) PEACHES & CREAM ICE CREAM - 10 Servings

8 ounces cream cheese, softened (16 grams)

211
Low Carb & No Carb Cookbook. (A) 130-Recipes. (B) 85-Low Carb Desserts. (C) 27-Restaurant Guide To Eating Out.

1 cup Splenda (24 grams)

2 eggs

1 tbsp lemon juice (1.3 grams)
1 tsp vanilla
2 1/2 cup heavy cream (24 grams) 1/2 cup diced peaches (9.4 grams)

212
Low Carb & No Carb Cookbook. (A) 130-Recipes. (B) 85-Low Carb Desserts. (C) 27-Restaurant Guide To Eating Out.

In a large mixer bowl beat cream cheese and Splenda smooth. Beat in the eggs, lemon juice, and vanilla until well combined. Stir in the cream and peaches. Freeze according to manufacturer's directions.

Carb Count: Recipe Total 64.7 grams, Per Serving 6.4 grams

(62)
<u>MINT ICE CREAM - 6 Serving</u>

4 egg yolks
3 cup heavy cream (28.8 grams)
1 tsp mint extract
2/3 cup Splenda (18 grams)

Combine half of the cream and mint extract in a saucepan. Bring to simmer. Remove from heat and let stand for 30 minutes. Mix in remaining cream. Beat the egg yolks and Splenda until pale yellow. Gradually beat in the cream mixture. Return mixture to

Low Carb & No Carb Cookbook. (A) 130-Recipes. (B) 85-Low Carb Desserts. (C) 27-Restaurant Guide To Eating Out.

saucepan and stir over medium heat until it thickens. Do not let the mixture boil. Chill. Once the mixture is cold, pour it into ice cream machine and freeze according to manufacturer's directions.

Carb Count: Recipe Total 46.8 grams, Per Serving 7.8 grams

(63) MACAROONS - 10 Servings

4 egg whites
1 1/4 cup Splenda (30 grams) 1/4 tsp salt
1/2 tsp vanilla extract (0.7 grams)
2 cup unsweetened shredded coconut (24.2 grams)

Beat egg whites until frothy. Stir in sweetener, salt, vanilla, and coconut. Spoon drop onto greased cookie sheet. Bake at 325 about 15 to 20 minutes, or until lightly browned.

Carb Count: Recipe Total 54.9 grams, Per Serving 5.4 grams

(64) GINGER COOKIES - 4 Servings

1/4 cup high gluten flour (6 grams)
2 eggs,

Low Carb & No Carb Cookbook. (A) 130-Recipes. (B) 85-Low Carb Desserts. (C) 27-Restaurant Guide To Eating Out.

separated
1/2 cup Splenda (12 grams)
1 tbsp heavy cream (0.5 grams)
1/2 tsp ground ginger

Beat egg whites until stiff. Add flour, Splenda, ginger and cream to yolks; beat until smooth. Fold in egg whites. Drop from teaspoon on a greased cookie sheet; flatten out, and bake at 325 degrees F for 20 minutes.

Carb Count: Recipe Total 18.5 grams, Per Serving 4.6 grams

(65) <u>CHOCOLATE MINTS - 10 Servings</u>

8 oz. Philadelphia cream cheese (16 grams)
1 cup butter
1/4 cup cocoa powder (11 grams)
1 tsp mint extract 1/4 cup cream (2.4 grams)
1/2 cup Splenda (12 grams) or to taste

Combine all ingredients. Roll into balls & refrigerate.

Carb Count: Recipe Total 31.4 grams, Per Serving 3.1 grams

(66) <u>COCOA BALLS- 12 Servings</u>

215
Low Carb & No Carb Cookbook. (A) 130-Recipes. (B) 85-Low Carb Desserts. (C) 27-Restaurant Guide To Eating Out.

1/2 cup sugar free peanut butter (24 grams; check your brand).
8 ounces cream cheese (16 grams)
1 tbsp heavy cream (0.6 grams)
2 tbsp almond extract
1/4 tsp salt
1/4 cup cocoa powder (11 grams)
1/4 cup chopped pecans (3.5 grams)
1/4 cup Splenda, or to taste (6 grams)

Combine all ingredients. Roll into balls & refrigerate.

Carb Count: Recipe Total 61.1 grams, Per Serving 5 grams

(67) SUGAR FREE GUMMY WORMS - 4 Servings

2 small packages sugar free jello
4 envelopes plain gelatin
1/2 cup water

Combine ingredients in a pan. Heat over medium heat until dissolved.
Pour into molds. Cool for twenty minutes.

Carb Count: Recipe Total 0 grams, Per Serving 0 grams

(68) PEANUT BUTTER BALLS - 6 Servings

1/3 cup chunky peanut butter (16 grams; check your brand)
1 tsp honey (3 grams)
1/2 tsp vanilla extract (0.7 grams)

216

Low Carb & No Carb Cookbook. (A) 130-Recipes. (B) 85-Low Carb Desserts. (C) 27-Restaurant Guide To Eating Out.

1/8 cup shredded coconut (3 grams)

Combine all above ingredients and mix well.
Form 12 balls and roll in coconut.
Refrigerate.

Carb Count: Recipe Total 22.7 grams, Per Serving 3.7 grams

(69) <u>FUDGE - 4 Servings</u>

2 oz unsweetened chocolate (8 grams)
1/2 cup Splenda, or to taste (12 grams)
4 tbsp butter
3 tbsp heavy cream (1.5 grams)
1/2 tsp vanilla (0.7 grams)

Combine all ingredients in pan over low heat.
Stir and until melted.
Pour into greased pan & chill.

Carb Count: Recipe Total 22.2 grams, Per Serving 5.5 grams

(70) <u>CINNAMON MERINGUES - 4 Servings</u>

2 egg whites
1/4 tsp
cream of
tartar dash
salt
1/2 cup Splenda (12 grams)
2 tsp ground cinnamon (3.6 grams)
1 tsp vanilla extract (1.5 grams)
1/2 tsp almond extract

Low Carb & No Carb Cookbook. (A) 130-Recipes. (B) 85-Low Carb Desserts. (C) 27-Restaurant Guide To Eating Out.

In medium bowl, combine egg whites with cream of tartar and salt; beat until soft peaks form. Fold in cinnamon, vanilla and almond extracts Drop by tablespoonfuls onto greased cookie sheets. Bake at 300 degrees F for 30 minutes.

Carb Count: Recipe Total 17.1 grams, Per Serving 4.2 grams

(71) PECAN COOKIES - 4 Servings

2 egg whites
2 cup crushed pecans (10 grams)
1 tbsp cinnamon (3.6 grams)
1/3 cup Splenda (8 grams)
1 tsp vanilla extract (1.5 grams)

Whip egg whites until frothy. Add remaining ingredients. Roll into balls, drop on grease cookie sheet. Cook for 15 minutes at 350 degrees F.

218

Low Carb & No Carb Cookbook. (A) 130-Recipes. (B) 85-Low Carb Desserts. (C) 27-Restaurant Guide To Eating Out.

Carb Count: Recipe Total 23.1 grams, Per Serving 5.7 grams

(72) **PEANUT BUTTER PECAN TREAT - 6 Servings**

3 tbsp butter
1/8 cup Splenda (3 grams)
2 cup ground pecans (10 grams)
1/2 cup Sugar free Peanut Butter (24 grams; check your brand).

Melt butter. Stir in Splenda and pecans. Spread on a cookie sheet & cook at 400 degrees for 10 minutes. While cooling, melt peanut butter and dip small batches of pecans in the melted peanut butter. Let harden & enjoy!

Carb Count: Recipe Total 37 grams, Per Serving 6.2 grams

(73) **FUDGSICLES - 4 Servings**

2 packages Sugar Free Cocoa Mix (8 grams)
1 cup cream (6.7 grams)
1/2 cup softened cream cheese
1 tsp vanilla

Dissolve cocoa mix in 1/2 cup of hot water. Add cream & cream cheese and mix well.
Pour into ice cube trays and freeze.

Carb Count: Recipe Total 14.7 grams, Per Serving 3.9 grams

219

Low Carb & No Carb Cookbook. (A) 130-Recipes. (B) 85-Low Carb Desserts. (C) 27-Restaurant Guide To Eating Out.

(74) <u>COCONUT CREAM - 4 Servings</u>

1 cup light cream (4.8 grams)
2 tbsp lemon juice (2.6 grams)
2 egg yolks
1 cup cottage cheese (6 grams) 1/4 cup Splenda (6 grams)
1/2 tsp coconut extract

Cream ingredients together and pour into greased pie dish. Bake at 300 degrees for 20 minutes.

Carb Count: Recipe Total 19.4 grams, Per Serving 4.85 grams

(75) <u>STRAWBERRY MERINGUE - 2 Servings</u>

2 egg whites
1/4 cup Splenda (6 grams)
1 cup strawberries (10.4 grams), crushed

Beat egg whites with Splenda until stiff. Fold in strawberries and chill.

Carb Count: Recipe Total 16.4 grams, Per Serving 8.2 grams

(76) <u>CHOCOLATE CUPCAKES - 10 Servings</u>

2 cup high gluten flour (24 grams)
1 cup Splendafi (24
   grams) 6 tbsp butter

220
Low Carb & No Carb Cookbook. (A) 130-Recipes. (B) 85-Low Carb Desserts. (C) 27-Restaurant Guide To Eating Out.

1/8 tsp cream of tartar

1 tsp vanilla e

221
Low Carb & No Carb Cookbook. (A) 130-Recipes. (B) 85-Low Carb Desserts. (C) 27-Restaurant Guide To Eating Out.

xtract

5 eggs, separated

2 tsp baking powder
1/4 cup cocoa (11 grams)

Preheat oven to 325EF. Whip egg whites with cream of tartar until stiff. In separate bowl, cream butter with egg yolks until fluffy. Add vanilla and Splendafi, beat until mixed. Add egg whites gradually & gently mix in. Add 1 cup of flour and fold in. Add remaining flour, baking powder and cocoa and fold in, being careful not to break down the egg whites. Fill greased muffin tins about half full. Bake at 325EF about 15 - 20 minutes.

222
Low Carb & No Carb Cookbook. (A) 130-Recipes. (B) 85-Low Carb Desserts. (C) 27-Restaurant Guide To Eating Out.

Carb Count: Recipe Total 59 grams, Per Serving 5.9 grams

(77) STRAWBERRY SHERBET - 5 Servings

2 cup strawberries, pureed (20 grams)
1/4 cup Splendafi (6 grams)
1 tbsp lemon juice (1.3 grams)
4 egg whites, beaten stiff

Mix strawberries with Splenda and lemon juice.. Fold the berries into the egg whites and mix thoroughly. Spoon into a plastic container and freeze for 4 hours.

Carb Count: Recipe Total 27.3 grams, Per Serving 5.4 grams

(78) LOW CARB TIRAMISU - 2 Servings

1/4 cup butter
1/4 cup heavy cream (2.4 grams)
2 large eggs
3/4 cup Splendafi (18 grams)
1/2 cup high gluten flour (6 grams)
1 tsp baking powder 1/4 cup flour (12 grams)
1/2 tsp vanilla extract (0.7 grams)

223
Low Carb & No Carb Cookbook. (A) 130-Recipes. (B) 85-Low Carb Desserts. (C) 27-Restaurant Guide To Eating Out.

Preheat oven to 375ЕF. In a small pan, heat the butter & cream. In a large bowl, beat eggs at high speed for several minutes. Add the 3/4 cup of Splenda and beat for 2 minutes. Add flours, baking powder, salt, vanilla & butter/cream mixture. Beat at low speed until smooth; pour into greased pan. Bake at 375ЕF for 15 minutes or until cakes springs back when lightly touched in the center. Cool completely. Serve with whipped cream (3.3 grams of carbs per cup).

Carb Count: Recipe Total 27.1 grams, Per Serving 13.5 grams

(79) SODA POP JELLO - 2 Serving

1 envelope plain gelatin
2 cups diet soda pop, any flavor

Soften gelatin with 1/2 cup soda. Bring to a boil, stirring constantly,
until gelatin dissolves. Add remaining soda and chill.

Carb Count: Recipe Total 0 grams, Per Serving 0 grams

(80) <u>ICEES</u>

224

Low Carb & No Carb Cookbook. (A) 130-Recipes. (B) 85-Low Carb Desserts. (C) 27-Restaurant Guide To Eating Out.

Freeze diet soda pop in ice cube trays. Crush & enjoy.

Carb Count: Recipe Total 0 grams, Per Serving 0 grams

(81) <u>CHOCOLATE RASPBERRY MOUSSE PIE - 8 Servings</u>

1 cup cream (9.4 grams)
1 cup water
1 package sugar free instant chocolate pudding mix (8 grams)
3/4 cup sour cream (12 grams)
1 cup whipped cream (3.3 grams)
1/2 cup raspberries (7.1 grams)

Beat cream & pudding mix until smooth. Add sour cream & topping, whisk until smooth. Fold in raspberries. Pour into pie pan. Sprinkle extra raspberries over top. Chill for 3 hours.

Carb Count: Recipe Total 39.8 grams, Per Serving 4.9 grams

(82) <u>PEACH PIE - 8 Servings</u>

1 can sliced peaches in juice, undrained (8 ounces), coarsely chopped (36 grams)
1 box fat free sugar free instant vanilla pudding mix (8 grams)
3/4
cup
sour

225
Low Carb & No Carb Cookbook. (A) 130-Recipes. (B) 85-Low Carb Desserts. (C) 27-Restaurant Guide To Eating Out.

cream (12 grams) 1/2 tsp vanilla (0.7 grams)
1/4 tsp cinnamon (0.5 grams)

In large bowl, combine all ingredients. Pour filing into pie pan. Chill for 3 hours.

Carb Count: Recipe Total 57.2 grams, Per Serving 7.1 grams

(83) CRISPY NUTS - 10 Servings

4 cup pecan pieces (40 grams)
2 tsp salt water

Mix nuts with salt and water and leave in a warm place overnight. Drain. Spread on a baking pan and heat at 150 degrees F for 12 hours, turning occasionally. Store in airtight container. Also good with walnuts.

Carb Count: Recipe Total 40 grams, Per Serving 4 grams

(84) PECAN PIE CRUST - 4 Servings

1 cup crispy pecans (10 grams)

226
Low Carb & No Carb Cookbook. (A) 130-Recipes. (B) 85-Low Carb Desserts. (C) 27-Restaurant Guide To Eating Out.

1/4 cup Splenda (6 grams)
1/4 tsp salt
1/2 cup butter, melted

Combine ingredients in food processor and combine until smooth. Place in buttered pie pan. Bake at 325 degrees F for 30 minutes. Can also use hazelnuts or almonds.

Carb Count: Recipe Total 16 grams, Per Serving 4 grams

(85) <u>COCONUT PIE CRUST - 4 Servings</u>

1/2 cup melted butter

227
Low Carb & No Carb Cookbook. (A) 130-Recipes. (B) 85-Low Carb Desserts. (C) 27-Restaurant Guide To Eating Out.

2 cup shredded unsweetened coconut (24.4 grams)

Mix coconut with butter. Press firmly into a buttered pie pan. Bake at 300 degrees F for 30 minutes until golden brown. Cool.

Carb Count: Recipe Total 24.4 grams, Per Serving 6 grams

INDEX
****
****

1. PECAN MERINGUES
2. LEMON MOUSSE
3. PINA COLADA ICEE
4. VANILLA ALMOND MOUSSE
5. CHOCOLATE RASPBERRY BROWNIES
6. VANILLA ALMOND COOKIES

228
Low Carb & No Carb Cookbook. (A) 130-Recipes. (B) 85-Low Carb Desserts. (C) 27-Restaurant Guide To Eating Out.

7. CHOCOLATE ANGEL FOOD CAKE
8. KEY LIME PIE
9. LOW-CARB FUDGE
10. CREAMY RASPBERRY JELLO
11. LIME PINEAPPLE CREAMY JELLO
12. LEMON CREPES
13. CHOCOLATE CREPES
14. BUTTERSCOTCH PUDDING
15. COCONUT CHOCOLATE PUDDING
16. TAPIOCA PUDDING
17. CHEWY COCONUT BARS
18. RASPBERRY BRULEE
19. PEACHES & RICOTTA
20. PEACH SOUFFLE
21. BROWNIE TORTE
22. CREAMY CAPPUCCINO
23. VANILLA CUSTARD
24. CHOCOLATE CHEESECAKE
25. STRAWBERRY CHEESECAKE
26. LEMON SHERBET
27. WALNUT TORTE
28. STRAWBERRIES & CREAM COOKIES
29. PEANUT BUTTER CHOCOLATE CUPS
30. RASPBERRY MERINGUES
31. BREAD PUDDING
32. CHOCOLATE PEANUT BUTTER PARFAITS
33. CHOCOLATE FROSTY
34. CHOCOLATE PEANUT BUTTER PIE
35. PEANUT BUTTER COOKIES
36. ZUCCHINI APPLES
37. CHOCOLATE CHEESE CAKE MUFFINS

229

Low Carb & No Carb Cookbook. (A) 130-Recipes. (B) 85-Low Carb Desserts. (C) 27-Restaurant Guide To Eating Out.

38. CHOCOLATE SHAKE
39. COFFEE & CREAM ICEE
40. SUGAR COOKIES
41. STRAWBERRY ICE CREAM
42. CHOCOLATE CAKE
43. CHOCOLATE FROSTING
44. CINNAMON PECAN MUFFINS
45. CINNAMON ROLLS
46. LOW CARB POPOVERS
47. VANILLA ICE CREAM
48. CHEESECAKE
49. LEMON ALMOND CAKE
50. FRENCH SILK PIE
51. CREME BRULEE
52. ORANGE CHOCOLATE CREAM
53. COCONUT CREME PIE
54. TIRAMISU
55. PEACHES AND CREAM
56. RASPBERRY ICE CREAM 57. PECAN ICE CREAM
58. CHOCOLATE ICE CREAM
59. PEANUT BUTTER ICE CREAM
60. COFFEE ICE CREAM
61. PEACHES & CREAM ICE CREAM
62. MINT ICE CREAM
63. MACAROONS
64. GINGER COOKIES
65. CHOCOLATE MINTS
66. COCOA BALLS
67. SUGAR FREE GUMMY WORMS
68. PEANUT BUTTER BALLS 69. FUDGE
70. CINNAMON MERINGUES

230

Low Carb & No Carb Cookbook. (A) 130-Recipes. (B) 85-Low Carb Desserts. (C) 27-Restaurant Guide To Eating Out.

71. PECAN COOKIES 72. PEANUT BUTTER PECAN TREAT
73. FUDGSICLES
74. COCONUT CREAM
75. STRAWBERRY MERINGUE
76. CHOCOLATE CUPCAKES
77. STRAWBERRY SHERBET
78. LOW CARB TIRAMISU
79. SODA POP JELLO
80. ICEES
81. CHOCOLATE RASPBERRY MOUSSE PIE
82. PEACH PIE
83. CRISPY NUTS
84. PECAN PIE CRUST
85. COCONUT PIE CRUST

LOW CARB RESTAURANT GUIDE TO EAT OUT

* Go to the restaurant with a firm and confident attitude that you only what you wish.

* When trying a new restaurant, call ahead to see if your special needs can be accommodated.

* Buffets can be dangerous. If you do go, simply pick your best protein choices and don't tempt yourself
  or rationalize choosing carbs.

231
Low Carb & No Carb Cookbook. (A) 130-Recipes. (B) 85-Low Carb Desserts. (C) 27-Restaurant Guide To Eating Out.

* Don't let your choices be swayed by other people, decide what YOU want and order it.

* Don't be afraid to ask for what you want - most restaurants are more than willing to accommodate you.

* If there is something on the table that is tempting you, ask that it be removed.

* If you do overeat carbs, continue with your eating plan as usual.

* Don't use little setbacks as an excuse to give up on your goals.

* Learn your weaknesses and avoid them.

APPLEBEE's®:

Applebee's only provides nutritional information for their low-fat dishes (and all are too high in carbs). I recommend these dishes as they all appear to be low carb. However, you may wish to wait until after induction to try them (you never know where hidden carbs are). I have put an asterisk by the meals that seem most appropriate for induction.

*APPLEBEE'S HOUSE SIRLOIN
A 9 oz. Sirloin served with steamed vegetables. Skip the new potatoes and Boboli® Oven Bread.

GRILLED SALMON
Char-broiled salmon fillet served with fresh steamed vegetables. Skip the rice pilaf and Boboli® Oven Bread.

CHICKEN OR STEAK FAJITAS
Skip the Tortillas

TEQUILA LIME CHICKEN
Substitute the rice with a house salad (no croutons).

*BOURBON STREET STEAK

232

Low Carb & No Carb Cookbook. (A) 130-Recipes. (B) 85-Low Carb Desserts. (C) 27-Restaurant Guide To Eating Out.

Ask for steamed veggies instead of the potatoes. Skip the bread.

RIBLET PLATTER
Substitute fries with a salad.

CHICKEN CAESAR SALAD
Skip the bread.

SANTA FE CHICKEN SALAD
Request no tortilla strips.

*BLACKENED CHICKEN SALAD
Skip the bread.

*HOUSE SALAD
Request no croutons.

*BUFFALO WINGS
Served with celery sticks & blue cheese dressing. Perfect low carb Appetizer

ARBY'S®:

Chicken Fingers
Calories: 290 Fat: 16 g Protein: 16 g Carbohydrates: 20 g

Side Salad
Calories: 23 Fat: 0 g Protein: 1 g Carbohydrates: 4 g

Garden Salad
Calories: 117 Fat: 2 g Protein: 9 g Carbohydrates: 16 g

Chef Salad
Calories: 205 Fat: 4 g Protein: 12 g Carbohydrates: 18 g

Chicken Salad
Calories: 204 Fat: 4 g Protein: 13 g Carbohydrates: 19 g

233
Low Carb & No Carb Cookbook. (A) 130-Recipes. (B) 85-Low Carb Desserts. (C) 27-Restaurant Guide To Eating Out.

Beef Soup, 6 oz.
Calories: 96 Fat: 3 g Protein: 5 g Carbohydrates: 14 g

Chicken Noodle Soup, 6 oz.
Calories :99 Fat: 2 g Protein: 6 g Carbohydrates: 15 g

Tomato Soup, 6 oz.
Calories: 84 Fat: 1 g Protein: 3 g Carbohydrates: 15 g

BLIMPIE'S®:

Blimpie's has recently introduced a new Carb-Counter menu with lots of great choices.

SANDWICHES –

Roast Beef, Cheddar (8 grams net carbs for 6" sandwich): Tender roast beef and real cheddar cheese
with lettuce, tomato and tangy wasabi sauce on 7-grain onion bread.

Turkey, Provolone (7 grams net carbs for 6" sandwich): Oven roasted turkey, provolone cheese, lettuce and tomato topped with FRENCH'S GourMayo (R) Southwestern Chipotle sauce on 7-grain onion bread.

Buffalo Chicken, Provolone Sun-Dried Tomato (8 grams net carbs for 6" sandwich): Tender sliced buffalo chicken topped with provolone, lettuce and tomato and finished with sun-dried tomato sauce on 7-grain onion bread.

Ham, Swiss (8.5 grams net carbs for 6" sandwich): 96% fat free ham with aged Swiss and yellow mustard
with tomato and lettuce on 7-grain onion bread.

SALADS –

Buffalo Chicken Salad (5 grams net carbs for standard size): 4 ounces of tangy buffalo chicken on a bed
of lettuce with rich bleu cheese dressing.

234
Low Carb & No Carb Cookbook. (A) 130-Recipes. (B) 85-Low Carb Desserts. (C) 27-Restaurant Guide To Eating Out.

Antipasto Salad (7 grams net carbs for standard size): Meats and cheeses from the BLIMPIE Best Sub
combined with fresh lettuce in this meat lover's salad.

SIDES –

Atkins Crunchers Chips (approximately 3 grams net carbs per bag): Available in Original Flavor, Nacho,
BBQ and Sour Cream.

DESSERT –

BLIMPIE Brownie (approximately 5 grams net carbs): A new version of BLIMPIE's popular dessert -
moist, chewy and absolutely delicious!

BEVERAGES –

SoBe Lean (1-gram net carb/no sugar for 8 oz. serving): A refreshing Cranberry-Grapefruit flavored
beverage with no Aspartame.

BOSTON MARKET®:

Skinless Rotisserie Turkey Breast
Cal: 170 Fat: 1 g Protein: 36 g Carbs: 1g

1/4 White Chicken, no skin or wing
Cal: 170 Fat: 4 g Protein: 33 g Carbs: 2g

1/4 White Meat Chicken with skin and wing
Cal: 280 Fat:12 g Protein: 40 g Carbs: 2g

1/4 Dark Meat Chicken, no skin
Cal: 190 Fat: 10g Protein: 22 g Carbs: 1g

1/4 Dark Meat Chicken with skin

235
Low Carb & No Carb Cookbook. (A) 130-Recipes. (B) 85-Low Carb Desserts. (C) 27-Restaurant Guide To Eating Out.

Cal: 320 Fat: 21g Protein: 30 g Carbs: 2g

Honey Glazed Ham (lean) 5 oz.
Cal: 210 Fat: 9 g Protein: 25 g Carbs: 9g

Meatloaf and Brown Gravy 7 oz.
Cal: 390 Fat: 22 g Protein: 30 g Carbs: 19 g

Chunky Chicken Salad 3/4 cup
Cal: 370 Fat: 27 g Protein: 28 g Carbs: 3g

Tabasco BBQ Drumstick
Cal: 130 Fat: 6 g Protein: 14 g Carbs: 4g

Tabasco BBQ Wing
Cal: 110 Fat: 7 g Protein: 2 g Carbs: 0g

Chicken Gravy
Cal: 231 Fat: 1 g Protein: 15 g Carbs: 4g

Creamed Spinach
Cal: 181 Fat: 20 g Protein: 11 g Carbs: 9g

Green Beans
Cal: 85 Fat: 6 g Protein: 1g Carbs: 5g

Caesar Side Salad
Cal: 113 Fat: 17 g Protein: 2g Carbs: 7g

Cucumber Salad
Cal: 136 Fat: 8 g Protein: 1g Carbs: 5g

Chicken Caesar Salad
Cal: 414 Fat: 12 g Protein: 24g Carbs: 3g

Fruit Salad 3/4 cup
Cal: 70 Fat: 0.5 g Protein: 1 g Carbs: 15 g

236
Low Carb & No Carb Cookbook. (A) 130-Recipes. (B) 85-Low Carb Desserts. (C) 27-Restaurant Guide To Eating Out.

Steamed Vegetables, 2/3 cup
Cal: 35 Fat: 0.5 g Protein: 2 g Carbs: 7 g

BURGER KING®:

Carb cutting tips:
Hold the Bun - order any BURGER KING® sandwich without the bun.
Skip the Ketchup - you'll save three grams of carbs per packet.
Avoid Sugar - drink diet soft drinks or water instead of regular sodas. Use sweetener in your coffee or tea,
or drink it plain.

Go Green - order a side salad instead of fries.

<u>Fire-Grilled Low Carb Bun-less Burgers, All 5g* of carbohydrates or less:</u>

Original WHOPPER® Sandwich

Original WHOPPER® Sandwich w/ cheese

DOUBLE WHOPPER® Sandwich

DOUBLE WHOPPER® Sandwich w/ cheese

WHOPPER JR.® Sandwich

WHOPPER JR.® Sandwich w/ cheese

BACON WHOPPER® Sandwich

BACON WHOPPER® Sandwich w/ cheese

Chicken WHOPPER® Sandwich

Served on a plate w/ a fork and knife
* excludes ketchup and mayo

237
Low Carb & No Carb Cookbook. (A) 130-Recipes. (B) 85-Low Carb Desserts. (C) 27-Restaurant Guide To Eating Out.

Many Burger King's no longer carry salads.

Chicken Salad
Cal: 142 Fat: 4 g Protein: 25 g Carbs: 10 g

Chef Salad
Cal: 178 Fat: 5 g Protein: 27 g Carbs: 12 g

Garden Salad
Cal: 95 Fat: 2 g Protein: 8 g Carbs: 10 g

Side Salad
Cal: 25 Fat: 0 g Protein: 1 g Carbs: 5 g

BK Broiler, meat only
Cal: 140 Fat: 4 g Protein: 21 g Carbs: 4g

CARL'S JR®:

Low Carb Six Dollar Burger
Calories: 690 Fat: 56 g Carbs: 6 g Protein: 31g

The Six Dollar Burger.
Calories: 956 Fat: 62 g Carbs: 61 g Protein: 38g

The Six Dollar Burger. (no bun)
Calories: 726 Fat: 59 g Carbs: 15 g Protein: 31g

Western Bacon Cheeseburger
Calories: 657 Fat: 31 g Carbs: 65 g Protein: 32 g

Western Bacon Cheeseburger
no bun, no BBQ sauce, no onion rings
Calories: 310 Fat: 24 g Carbs: 1 g Protein: 23 g

BBQ Sauce
Calories: 48 Fat: 0 g Carbs: 11 g Protein: 1 g

Low Carb & No Carb Cookbook. (A) 130-Recipes. (B) 85-Low Carb Desserts. (C) 27-Restaurant Guide To Eating Out.

Larger Bun (Western Bacon Cheeseburger)
Calories: 222 Fat: 3 g Carbs: 43 g Protein: 7 g

Onion Rings (on Western Bacon Cheeseburger)
Calories: 77 Fat: 4 g Carbs: 10 g Protein: 1 g

Famous Star Hamburger, no bun, no special sauce
Calories: 410 Fat: 35 g Carbs: 4 g Protein: 20 g

Special sauce
Calories: 19 Fat: 0 g Carbs: 4 g Protein: 0 g

Spicy Chicken Sandwich, no bun, no tomatoes (2 g of carbs)
Calories: 313 Fat: 24 g Carbs: 14 g Protein: 8 g

Hamburger
Calories: 284 Fat: 9 g Carbs: 36 g Protein: 14 g

Hamburger, no bun
Calories: 120 Fat: 7 g Carbs: 4 g Protein: 9 g

Hamburger bun
Calories: 164 Fat: 2 g Carbs: 32 g Protein: 5 g

Double Chili Cheese Burger, no bun
Calories: 732 Fat: 53 g Carbs: 14 g Protein: 52 g

Double Chili Cheese Burger, no bun, no tomatoes
Calories: 720 Fat: 53 g Carbs: 12 g Protein: 52 g

Chicken Tenders, 5
Cal: 230 Fat: 14 g Protein: 14 g Carbs: 11 g

Chicken Stars, 6
Cal: 280 Fat: 19 g Protein: 12 g Carbs: 15 g

Ranch Dipping Sauce
Cal: 170 Fat: 17 g Protein: 0 g Carbs: 2 g

239
Low Carb & No Carb Cookbook. (A) 130-Recipes. (B) 85-Low Carb Desserts. (C) 27-Restaurant Guide To Eating Out.

BBQ Dipping Sauce
Cal: 9 Fat: 0 g Protein: 0 g Carbs: 9 g

Sweet n Sour Dipping Sauce
Cal: 45 Fat: 0 g Protein: 0 g Carbs: 11 g

Charbroiled Chicken Salad
Cal: 200 Fat: 7 g Protein: 25 g Carbs: 12 g

Chicken Stars, 6 pieces
Cal: 256 Fat: 16 g Protein: 13 g Carbs: 14 g

Garden Salad to-go
Cal: 50 Fat: 2.5 g Protein: 3 g Carbs: 1 g

Scrambled Eggs
Cal:160 Fat: 11 g Protein: 13 g Carbs: 1 g

Bacon, 2 strips
Cal: 50 Fat: 4 g Protein: 39 g Carbs: 0 g

Blue Cheese Dressing
Cal: 324 Fat: 35 g Protein: 2 g Carbs: 1 g

Ranch Dressing
Cal: 315 Fat: 35 g Protein: 2 g Carbs: 1 g

Fat Free Italian Dressing
Cal: 15 Fat: 0 g Protein: 0 g Carbs: 4g

CHICK-FIL-A®:

Hearty Breast of Chicken Soup (cup)
Cal: 110 Fat: 2 g Protein: 16 g Carbs: 10 g

Chargrilled Chicken Garden Salad
Cal: 170 Fat: 3 g Protein: 26 g Carbs: 10 g

240

Low Carb & No Carb Cookbook. (A) 130-Recipes. (B) 85-Low Carb Desserts. (C) 27-Restaurant Guide To Eating Out.

Chik-n Strips (4)
Cal: 230 Fat: 8 g Protein: 29 g Carbs: 10 g

Chik-n Nuggets (8)
Cal: 290 Fat: 14 g Protein: 29 g Carbs: 12 g

Chik-n Strips Salad
Cal: 240 Fat: 10 g Protein: 30 g Carbs: 7 g

Chicken Caesar Salad
Cal: 170 Fat: 10 g Protein: 34 g Carbs: 1 g

Side Salad
Cal: 80 Fat: 4.5 g Protein: 26 g Carbs: 6 g

Cole Slaw (cup)
Cal: 79 Fat: 6 g Protein: 5 g Carbs: 11g

BBQ Sauce
Cal: 45 Fat: 0 g Protein: 0 g Carbs: 11 g

Honey Mustard Sauce
Cal: 45 Fat: 0 g Protein: 0 g Carbs: 11 g

Dijon
Cal: 60 Fat: 5 g Protein: 0 g Carbs: 2 g

Polynesian Sauce
Cal: 110 Fat: 6 g Protein: 0 g Carbs: 13 g

Light Italian
Cal: 20 Fat: 0.5 g Protein: 0 g Carbs: 3 g

Fat Free Dijon Mustard
Cal: 60 Fat: 0 g Protein: 0 g Carbs: 14 g

House Dressing

241
Low Carb & No Carb Cookbook. (A) 130-Recipes. (B) 85-Low Carb Desserts. (C) 27-Restaurant Guide To Eating Out.

Cal: 210 Fat: 17 g Protein: 0 g Carbs: 9 g

Spicy Dressing
Cal: 210 Fat: 22 g Protein: 0 g Carbs: 2 g

Blue Cheese Dressing
Cal: 190 Fat: 20 g Protein: 0 g Carbs: 2 g
Buttermilk Ranch Dressing Cal: 190 Fat: 20 g Protein: 1 g Carbs: 2 g

Basil Vinaigrette
Cal: 210 Fat: 21 g Protein: 0 g Carbs: 4 g

Ice Cream Cone, small
Cal: 140 Fat: 4 g Protein: 11 g Carbs: 16 g

Lemon Pie
Cal: 280 Fat: 22 g Protein: 1 g Carbs: 19 g

Chili's®:

Chili's is now offering a low carb menu

GRILL

Ribeye Steak
Carbs: 8 g Fiber: 4 g Net Carbs: 4 g

Monterey Chicken
Carbs: 24 g Fiber: 6 g Net Carbs: 18 g

Grilled Salmon
Carbs: 11 g Fiber: 4 g Net Carbs: 7 g

Chicken or Steak Fajitas
Carbs: 17 g Fiber:10 g Net Carbs: 7 g

Mushroom Jack Fajitas

242

Low Carb & No Carb Cookbook. (A) 130-Recipes. (B) 85-Low Carb Desserts. (C) 27-Restaurant Guide To Eating Out.

Carbs: 24 g Fiber: 11 g Net Carbs: 13 g

APPETIZERS –

Buffalo Wings
Carbs: 2 g Fiber: 3 g Net Carbs: 0 g

SALADS –

Fajita Caesar
Carbs: 11 g Fiber: 4 g Net Carbs: 7 g

Dinner Salad
Carbs: 8 g Fiber: 3 g Net Carbs: 5 g

Dinner Caesar Salad
Carbs: 5 g Fiber: 2 g Net Carbs: 0 g

SOUPS–

Beef Chili
Carbs: 25 g Fiber: 6 g Net Carbs: 19 g

Broccoli Cheese
Carbs: 20 g Fiber: 2 g Net Carbs: 18 g

BUN-LESS BURGERS –

Old Timer Burger
Carbs: 11 g Fiber: 6 g Net Carbs: 5 g

Bacon Burger
Carbs: 9 g Fiber: 6 g Net Carbs: 3 g

Mushroom Burger
Carbs: 14 g Fiber: 6 g Net Carbs: 8 g

DENNY'S®:

243

Low Carb & No Carb Cookbook. (A) 130-Recipes. (B) 85-Low Carb Desserts. (C) 27-Restaurant Guide To Eating Out.

Garden Salad Deluxe with Chicken
Cal: 264 Fat: 11 g Protein: 32 g Carbs: 10 g

Garden Salad Deluxe with Salmon
Cal: 389 Fat: 9 g Protein: 67 g Carbs: 10 g

Garden Salad Deluxe with Turkey & Ham
Cal: 322 Fat: 11 g Protein: 43 g Carbs: 10g

Vegetable Beef Soup, 8 oz.
Cal: 79 Fat: 1 g Protein: 6 g Carbs: 11 g

Chicken Noodle Soup, 8 oz.
Cal: 60 Fat: 2 g Protein: 2 g Carbs: 8 g

Pot Roast with Gravy
Cal: 292 Fat: 11 g Protein: 42 g Carbs: 5 g

Grilled Chicken Dinner, no sides
Cal: 130 Fat: 4 g Protein: 24 g Carbs: 0 g

Alaskan Salmon Dinner, no sides
Cal: 210 Fat: 4 g Protein: 43 g Carbs: 1 g

2 eggs
Cal: 120 Fat:10 g Protein: 6 Carbs: 0g

Egg beaters, 2 Servings
Cal: 71 Fat: 5 g Protein: 5 g Carbs: 1 g

Broccoli in butter
Cal: 50 Fat: 2 g Protein: 3 g Carbs: 7 g

Carrots in honey glaze
Cal: 80 Fat: 2 g Protein: 1 g Carbs: 12 g

Corn in butter

Low Carb & No Carb Cookbook. (A) 130-Recipes. (B) 85-Low Carb Desserts. (C) 27-Restaurant Guide To Eating Out.

Cal: 120 Fat: 4 g Protein: 2 g Carbs: 19 g

Green peas in butter
Cal: 100 Fat: 2 g Protein: 5 g Carbs: 14 g

Green beans with bacon
Cal: 60 Fat: 4 g Protein: 1 g Carbs: 6 g

Fat Free Honey Mustard Dressing
Cal: 38 Fat: 0 g Protein:0 g Carbs: 9 g

DOMINO'S PIZZA®:

Barbeque Buffalo Wings, 1 pc
Cal: 50 Fat: 2.4 g Protein: 6 g Carbs: 2 g

Hot Buffalo Wings, 1 pc
Cal: 45 Fat: 2.4 g Protein: 6 g Carbs: 1 g

Breadsticks, 1
Cal: 78 Fat: 3 g Protein: 2 g Carbs: 11 g

Cheesy Bread
Cal: 103 Fat: 5 g Protein: 3 g Carbs: 11 g

Large Garden Salad
Cal: 39 Fat: 0 g Protein: 2 g Carbs: 8 g

Small Garden Salad
Cal: 22 Fat: 0 g Protein: 1 g Carbs: 4 g

Blue Cheese Dressing
Cal: 220 Fat: 24 g Protein: 0 g Carbs: 2 g

Creamy Caesar Dressing
Cal: 200 Fat: 22 g Protein: 0 g Carbs: 2 g

245
Low Carb & No Carb Cookbook. (A) 130-Recipes. (B) 85-Low Carb Desserts. (C) 27-Restaurant Guide To Eating Out.

Fat Free Ranch Dressing
Cal: 40 Fat: 0 g Protein: 0 g Carbs: 10 g

Italian Dressing
Cal: 220 Fat: 24 g Protein: 0 g Carbs: 1 g

EL POLLO LOCO®:

Chicken Soft Taco
Cal: 237 Fat: 12 g Protein: 17 g Carbs: 15 g

Taco Al Carbon
Cal: 164 Fat: 6 g Protein: 14 g Carbs: 13 g

Chicken Breast, Flame Broiled
Cal: 160 Fat: 6 g Protein: 26 g Carbs: 0 g

Chicken Wing, Flame Broiled
Cal: 110 Fat: 6 g Protein: 12 g Carbs: 0 g

Chicken Leg, Flame Broiled
Cal: 90 Fat: 5 g Protein: 11 g Carbs: 0 g

Chicken Thigh, Flame Broiled
Cal: 180 Fat: 12 g Protein: 16 g Carbs: 0 g

4.5 Corn Tortilla
Cal: 32 Fat: 0.5 g Protein: 1 g Carbs: 6 g

6 Corn Tortilla
Cal: 70 Fat: 1 g Protein: 1 g Carbs: 14 g

6.5 Flour Tortilla
Cal: 90 Fat: 3 g Protein: 3 g Carbs: 13 g

Garden Salad, regular
Cal: 105 Fat: 7 g Protein: 5 g Carbs: 7 g

246
Low Carb & No Carb Cookbook. (A) 130-Recipes. (B) 85-Low Carb Desserts. (C) 27-Restaurant Guide To Eating Out.

Corn on the Cob
Cal: 80 Fat: 1 g Protein: 3 g Carbs: 18 g

Cole Slaw
Cal: 206 Fat: 16 g Protein: 2 g Carbs: 12 g

Mashed Potatoes
Cal: 97 Fat: 1 g Protein: 3 g Carbs: 21 g

Gravy
Cal: 14 Fat: 1 g Protein: 0 g Carbs: 2 g

Fresh Vegetables
Cal: 57 Fat: 2 g Protein: 2 g Carbs: 8 g

Sour Cream, Light
Cal: 45 Fat: 2 g Protein: 2 g Carbs: 3 g

Guacamole
Cal: 20 Fat: 2 g Protein: 0 g Carbs: 3 g

Jalapeno Hot Sauce, 1 pkt
Cal: 5 Fat: 0 g Protein: 0 g Carbs: 1 g

House Salsa
Cal: 6 Fat: 0 g Protein: 0 g Carbs: 1 g

Pico de Gallo Salsa
Cal: 11 Fat: 0.5 g Protein: 0 g Carbs: 1.5 g

Spicy Chipotle Salsa
Cal: 7 Fat: 0 g Protein: 0 g Carbs: 1 g

Avocado Salsa
Cal: 12 Fat: 1 g Protein: 0 g Carbs: 1 g

Light Italian Salad Dressing

247
Low Carb & No Carb Cookbook. (A) 130-Recipes. (B) 85-Low Carb Desserts. (C) 27-Restaurant Guide To Eating Out.

Cal: 25 Fat: 1 g Protein: 0 g Carbs: 3 g

Ranch Dressing
Cal: 350 Fat: 39 g Protein: 0 g Carbs: 2 g

1,000 Island Dressing
Cal: 270 Fat: 27 g Protein: 1 g Carbs: 9 g

Blue Cheese Dressing
Cal: 300 Fat: 32 g Protein: 2 g Carbs: 2 g

Creamy Cilantro Dressing
Cal: 266 Fat: 29 g Protein: 0 g Carbs: 1 g

Southwest Dressing
Cal: 301 Fat: 32 g Protein: 0 g Carbs: 2 g

HARDEE'S®:

SANDWICHES
½ pound Sour Dough, bun-less
Cal: 813 Fat: 71 g Protein: 36 g Carbs: 4 g

½ pound Six Dollar, bun-less
Cal: 620 Fat: 48 g Protein: 32 g Carbs: 10 g

Slammer, bun-less
Cal: 141 Fat: 42 g Protein: 15 g Carbs: 1.1 g

1/3 lb. Bacon Cheeseburger, bun-less
Cal: 505 Fat: 32 g Protein: 24 g Carbs: 1.1 g

1/3 lb. Cheeseburger, bun-less
Cal: 432 Fat: 36 g Protein: 29 g Carbs: 1.1 g

1/3 lb. Thickburger, bun-less
Cal: 450 Fat: 36 g Protein: 28 g Carbs: 1.1 g

248

Low Carb & No Carb Cookbook. (A) 130-Recipes. (B) 85-Low Carb Desserts. (C) 27-Restaurant Guide To Eating Out.

1/3 lb. Mushroom Swiss Thickburger, bun-less
Cal: 487 Fat: 39 g Protein: 28 g Carbs: 1.1 g

2/3 lb. Double Bacon Cheeseburger, bun-less
Cal: 899 Fat: 75 g Protein: 20 g Carbs: 1.1 g

Big Chicken Fillet, bun-less
Cal: 367 Fat: 15 g Protein: 15 g Carbs: 1.1 g

Big Hot Ham-n-Cheese, bun-less
Cal: 306 Fat: 19 g Protein: 15 g Carbs: 1.1 g

Big Roast Beef Sandwich, bun-less
Cal: 260 Fat: 18 g Protein: 28 g Carbs: 1.1 g

Roast Beef Sandwich, bun-less
Cal: 174 Fat: 12 g Protein: 19 g Carbs: 1.1 g

Charbroiled Chicken Sandwich, bun-less
Cal: 196 Fat: 3 g Protein: 35 g Carbs: 1.1 g

Spicy Chicken Sandwich, bun-less
Cal: 198 Fat: 2 g Protein: 13 g Carbs: 1.1 g

SALADS –

Garden Salad
Cal: 220 Fat: 13 g Protein: 12 g Carbs: 11 g

Grilled Chicken Salad
Cal: 150 Fat: 3 g Protein: 20 g Carbs: 11 g

Side Salad
Cal: 25 Fat: 0 g Protein: 1 g Carbs: 4 g

SIDES –

249
Low Carb & No Carb Cookbook. (A) 130-Recipes. (B) 85-Low Carb Desserts. (C) 27-Restaurant Guide To Eating Out.

Fried Chicken Breast
Cal: 317 Fat: 15 g Protein: 29 g Carbs: 29 g

Fried Chicken Leg
Cal: 170 Fat: 7 g Protein: 13 g Carbs: 15 g

Coleslaw (1/2 cup)
Cal: 240 Fat: 20 g Protein: 2 g Carbs: 13 g

Mashed Potatoes (1/2 cup)
Cal:70 Fat: 0 g Protein: 2 g Carbs: 14 g

Gravy
Cal: 20 Fat: 0 g Protein: 0 g Carbs: 3 g

IHOP®:

Buckwheat Pancake, 1 ea.
Cal: 110 Fat: 4 g Protein: 3 g Carbs: 15 g

Buttermilk Pancake, 1 ea.
Cal: 110 Fat: 3 g Protein: 3 g Carbs: 17 g

Country Griddle Pancake, 1 ea.
Cal: 120 Fat: 3.5 g Protein: 3 g Carbs: 19 g

Egg Crepe, 1 ea.
Cal: 120 Fat: 6 g Protein: 3 g Carbs: 14 g

Harvest Grain 'N Nut Pancake, 1 ea.
Cal: 180 Fat: 9 g Protein: 5 g Carbs: 20 g

Scrambled eggs, 2
Cal: 125 Fat:10 g Protein: 6.5 g Carbs: 0 g

Bacon, 2 strips
Cal: 50 Fat: 4 g Protein: 39 g Carbs: 0 g

250
Low Carb & No Carb Cookbook. (A) 130-Recipes. (B) 85-Low Carb Desserts. (C) 27-Restaurant Guide To Eating Out.

IN-N-OUT BURGER®:

Hamburger, Protein style, with onions
Cal: 240 Fat: 17 g Protein: 13 g Carbs: 11 g

Cheeseburger, Protein style, with onions
Cal: 330 Fat: 25 g Protein: 18 g Carbs: 11 g

Double-Double, Protein style, with onions
Cal: 520 Fat: 39 g Protein: 33 g Carbs: 11 g

JACK IN THE BOX®:

Option: Order hamburgers or cheeseburgers and discard the bun.

Chicken Fajita Pita
Cal: 280 Fat: 9 g Protein: 24 g Carbs: 22 g

Taco
Cal: 170 Fat: 10 g Protein: 7 g Carbs: 12 g

Taco Monster
Cal: 270 Fat: 19 g Protein: 12 g Carbs: 19 g

Chicken Salad
Cal: 200 Fat: 9 g Protein: 24 g Carbs: 8 g

Side Salad
Cal: 50 Fat: 3 g Protein: 2 g Carbs: 3 g

KENNY ROGER'S ROASTERS®:

Chicken Caesar Salad
Cal: 285 Fat: 9 g Protein: 34 g Carbs: 18 g

Roasted Chicken Salad

251
Low Carb & No Carb Cookbook. (A) 130-Recipes. (B) 85-Low Carb Desserts. (C) 27-Restaurant Guide To Eating Out.

Cal: 292 Fat: 10 g Protein: 35 g Carbs: 19 g

Soup, Chicken Noodle, cup
Cal: 55 Fat: 1 g Protein: 4 g Carbs: 7 g

Soup, Chicken Noodle, bowl
Cal: 91 Fat: 2 g Protein: 7 g Carbs: 12 g

1/4 Chicken, white w/o skin
Cal: 144 Fat: 2 g Protein: 32 g Carbs: 0 g

1/2 Chicken, w/o skin
Cal: 313 Fat: 10 g Protein: 56 g Carbs: 1 g

Sliced Turkey Breast, 4.5 oz.
Cal: 158 Fat: 2 g Protein: 38 g Carbs: 0 g

Corn on the Cob, 2.25 oz.
Cal: 68 Fat: 1 g Protein: 2 g Carbs: 14 g

Steamed Vegetables, 4.25 oz.
Cal: 48 Fat: 0 g Protein: 3 g Carbs: 8 g

Tomato Cucumber Salad 6
Cal: 123 Fat: 2 g Protein: 1 g Carbs: 10 g

Side Salad, 4.73 oz.
Cal: 23 Fat: 0 g Protein: 1 g Carbs: 5 g

Fat Free Italian Dressing
Cal: 35 Fat: 0 g Protein: 0 g Carbs: 8 g

KFC®:

Tender Roast Chicken Breast w/skin
Cal: 251 Fat: 11 g Protein: 37 g Carbs: 1 g

Tender Roast Chicken Breast w/o skin

Cal: 169 Fat: 4 g Protein: 31 g Carbs: 1 g

Tender Roast Chicken Drumstick w/skin
Cal: 97 Fat: 4 g Protein: 15 g Carbs: 0 g

Tender Roast Chicken Drumstick w/o skin
Cal: 67 Fat: 2 g Protein: 11 g Carbs: 0 g

Tender Roast Chicken Thigh w/skin
Cal: 207 Fat: 6 g Protein: 18 g Carbs: 1 g

Tender Roast Chicken Thigh w/o skin
Cal: 106 Fat: 12 g Protein: 13 g Carbs: 0 g

Tender Roast Chicken Wing w/skin
Cal: 121 Fat: 8 g Protein: 12 g Carbs: 1 g

Original Recipe Chicken Breast
Cal: 400 Fat: 24 g Protein: 29 g Carbs: 16 g

Original Recipe Chicken Drumstick
Cal:140 Fat: 9 g Protein: 13 g Carbs: 4 g

Original Recipe Chicken Thigh
Cal: 250 Fat: 18 g Protein: 16 g Carbs: 6 g

Original Recipe Chicken Wing
Cal:140 Fat:10 g Protein: 9 g Carbs: 5 g

Hot and Spicy Chicken Breast
Cal: 530 Fat: 35 g Protein: 32 g Carbs: 23 g

Hot and Spicy Chicken Drumstick
Cal:190 Fat: 11 g Protein: 13 g Carbs: 10 g

Hot and Spicy Chicken Thigh
Cal: 370 Fat: 27 g Protein: 18 g Carbs: 13 g

253
Low Carb & No Carb Cookbook. (A) 130-Recipes. (B) 85-Low Carb Desserts. (C) 27-Restaurant Guide To Eating Out.

Hot and Spicy Chicken Wing
Cal:210 Fat: 15 g Protein: 10 g Carbs: 9 g

Colonel's Crispy Strips, 3
Cal:261 Fat: 16 g Protein: 20 g Carbs: 10 g

Green Beans
Cal: 45 Fat: 2 g Protein: 1 g Carbs: 7 g

Mean Greens
Cal: 70 Fat: 3 g Protein: 4 g Carbs: 11 g

Mashed Potatoes with Gravy
Cal: 120 Fat: 6 g Protein: 1 g Carbs: 17 g

LITTLE CAESAR'S®:

Chicken Wings
Cal: 50 Fat: 14 g Protein: 4 g Carbs: 15 g

Pan Cheese Pizza, 1 slice
Cal: 160 Fat: 6 g Protein: 7 g Carbs: 20 g

Pan Pepperoni Pizza, 1 slice
Cal: 170 Fat: 7 g Protein: 8 g Carbs: 20 g

Pepperoni Pizza, 1 slice
Cal: 220 Fat: 9 g Protein: 11 g Carbs: 23 g

Antipasto Salad
Cal: 80 Fat: 6 g Protein: 5 g Carbs: 4 g

Caesar Salad
Cal: 80 Fat: 3 g Protein: 5 g Carbs: 7 g

Greek Salad

Low Carb & No Carb Cookbook. (A) 130-Recipes. (B) 85-Low Carb Desserts. (C) 27-Restaurant Guide To Eating Out.

Cal: 60 Fat: 3 g Protein: 3 g Carbs: 5 g

Tossed Salad
Cal: 50 Fat: 0 g Protein: 2 g Carbs:9 g

Fat Free Italian Salad Dressing
Cal: 25 Fat: 0 g Protein: 0 g Carbs: 5 g

Ranch Dressing
Cal: 270 Fat: 29 g Protein: 0 g Carbs: 1 g

1,000 Island Dressing
Cal: 220 Fat: 21 g Protein: 0 g Carbs: 7 g

Blue Cheese Dressing
Cal: 230 Fat: 24 g Protein: 2 g Carbs: 2 g

Creamy Caesar Dressing
Cal: 220 Fat: 23 g Protein: 1 g Carbs: 2 g

Honey French Dressing
Cal: 220 Fat: 18 g Protein: 0 g Carbs: 14 g

LONG JOHN SILVER'S®:

Grilled Chicken Salad
Cal: 140 Fat: 3 g Protein: 20 g Carbs: 10 g

Garden Salad
Cal: 45 Fat:0 g Protein: 3 g Carbs: 9 g

Ocean Chef Salad
Cal: 130 Fat: 2 g Protein: 15 g Carbs: 14 g

Fat Free French Dressing
Cal: 40 Fat:0 g Protein: 0 g Carbs: 10 g

Ranch Dressing

255
Low Carb & No Carb Cookbook. (A) 130-Recipes. (B) 85-Low Carb Desserts. (C) 27-Restaurant Guide To Eating Out.

Cal: 170 Fat: 18 g Protein: 0 g Carbs: 1 g

1,000 Island Dressing
Cal: 120 Fat: 10 g Protein: 0 g Carbs: 5 g

Fat Free Ranch Dressing
Cal: 40 Fat: 0 g Protein: 0 g Carbs: 9 g

Italian Dressing
Cal: 90 Fat: 9 g Protein: 0 g Carbs: 2 g

Battered Chicken Plank
Cal: 140 Fat: 8 g Protein: 8 g Carbs: 9 g

Battered Shrimp
Cal: 45 Fat: 3 g Protein: 2 g Carbs: 3 g

Lemon Crumb Fish, 2 pieces
Cal: 240 Fat: 8 g Protein: 23 g Carbs: 9 g

Battered Fish, regular
Cal: 230 Fat: 13 g Protein: 12 g Carbs: 16 g

Flavor baked Chicken, 1 piece
Cal: 110 Fat: 3 g Protein: 15 g Carbs: 1 g

Flavor baked Fish, 1 piece
Cal: 90 Fat: 3 g Protein: 14 g Carbs: 1 g

Green Beans
Cal: 30 Fat: 0 g Protein: 1 g Carbs: 6 g

Side Salad
Cal: 25 Fat: 0 g Protein: 1 g Carbs: 5 g

Broccoli Cheese Soup
Cal: 180 Fat: 12 g Protein: 5 g Carbs: 13 g

256

Low Carb & No Carb Cookbook. (A) 130-Recipes. (B) 85-Low Carb Desserts. (C) 27-Restaurant Guide To Eating Out.

Hush Puppy
Cal: 60 Fat: 3 g Protein: 1 g Carbs: 9 g

Tartar Sauce
Cal: 40 Fat: 4 g Protein: 0 g Carbs: 2 g

Malt Vinegar
Cal: 0 Fat: 0 g Protein: 0 g Carbs: 0 g

Sweet n Sour Sauce
Cal: 20 Fat: 0 g Protein: 0 g Carbs: 5 g

Honey Mustard Sauce
Cal: 20 Fat: 0 g Protein: 0 g Carbs: 5 g

Shrimp Sauce
Cal: 15 Fat: 0 g Protein: 0 g Carbs: 3 g

MCDONALD'S®:

Scrambled Eggs
Cal: 160 Fat: 1 g Protein: 13 g Carbs: 1 g

Egg McMuffin
Cal: 290 Fat: 12 g Protein: 27 g Carbs: 17 g

Egg McMuffin, no bread
Cal:161 Fat: 11 g Protein: 13 g Carbs: 2 g

Sausage McMuffin, no bread
Cal:311 Fat: 27 g Protein: 15 g Carbs: 2 g

Breakfast Burrito
Cal:290 Fat: 16 g Protein: 24 g Carbs: 13 g

Grilled Chicken, meat only
Cal: 121 Fat: 3 g Protein: 19 g Carbs: 4 g

257
Low Carb & No Carb Cookbook. (A) 130-Recipes. (B) 85-Low Carb Desserts. (C) 27-Restaurant Guide To Eating Out.

Hamburger patty
Cal: 102 Fat: 8 g Protein: 7 g Carbs: 0 g

Cheese
Cal: 52 Fat: 4 g Protein: 3 g Carbs: 0 g

Quarter Pounder, meat only
Cal: 234 Fat: 18 g Protein: 18 g Carbs: 0 g

Crispy Chicken, meat only
Cal: 222 Fat: 12 g Protein: 16 g Carbs: 13 g

Fish patty
Cal: 152 Fat: 6 g Protein: 15 g Carbs: 0 g

Tartar sauce
Cal: 145 Fat: 14 g Protein: 0g Carbs: 1 g

Chicken Nuggets, 4 pieces
Cal: 190 Fat: 11 g Protein: 10 g Carbs: 13 g

Onion on sandwiches
Cal: 11 Fat: 0 g Protein: 0 g Carbs: 3 g

Lettuce on sandwiches
Cal: 3 Fat: 0 g Protein: 0 g Carbs: 1 g

Mayo on sandwiches
Cal: 104 Fat: 11 g Protein: 0 g Carbs: 0 g

Tomato on sandwiches
Cal: 5 Fat: 0 g Protein: 0 g Carbs: 1 g

Grill Seasoning (upon request)
Cal: 0 Fat: 0 g Protein: 0 g Carbs: 3 g

258

Low Carb & No Carb Cookbook. (A) 130-Recipes. (B) 85-Low Carb Desserts. (C) 27-Restaurant Guide To Eating Out.

Chunky Chicken Salad
Cal: 150 Fat: 4 g Protein: 25 g Carbs: 7 g

Fajita Chicken Salad
Cal: 160 Fat: 6 g Protein: 9 g Carbs: 20 g

Chef McShaker
Cal: 150 Fat: 8 g Protein: 17 g Carbs: 5 g

Garden McShaker
Cal: 100 Fat: 6 g Protein: 7 g Carbs: 4 g

Chicken Caesar McShaker
Cal: 150 Fat: 8 g Protein: 17 g Carbs: 5 g

Grilled Chicken Caesar Salad
Cal: 150 Fat: 13 g Protein: 17 g Carbs: 5 g

Garden Salad
Cal: 80 Fat: 4 g Protein: 7 g Carbs: 6 g

Side Salad
Cal:30 Fat: 1 g Protein: 2 g Carbs: 4 g

Lite Vinaigrette (1 pkg)
Cal: 50 Fat: 2 g Protein: 0 g Carbs: 9 g

Fat Free Herb Vinaigrette (1 pkg)
Cal: 35 Fat: 0 g Protein: 0 g Carbs: 8 g

Hot Mustard Sauce (1 pkg)
Cal: 60 Fat: 3.5 g Protein: 1g Carbs: 7 g

Barbeque Sauce (1 pkg)
Cal: 45 Fat: 0 g Protein: 0 g Carbs: 10 g

Sweet 'N Sour Sauce (1 pkg)
Cal: 50 Fat: 0 g Protein: 0 g Carbs: 11 g

259
Low Carb & No Carb Cookbook. (A) 130-Recipes. (B) 85-Low Carb Desserts. (C) 27-Restaurant Guide To Eating Out.

Honey (1 pkg)
Cal: 45 Fat: 0 g Protein: 0 g Carbs: 11 g

Honey Mustard (1 pkg)
Cal: 50 Fat: 4.5 g Protein: 0 g Carbs: 10 g

Light Mayo (1 pkg)
Cal: 40 Fat: 4 g Protein: 0 g Carbs: <1 g

Ketchup
Cal: 13 Fat: 0 g Protein: 0 g Carbs: 3 g

Mustard
Cal: 1 Fat: 0 g Protein: 0 g Carbs: 0 g

PIZZA HUT®:

The Edge Chicken Veggie, 1 slice
Cal: 120 Fat: 3 g Protein: 6 g Carbs: 16 g

The Edge Taco, 1 slice
Cal: 140 Fat: 5 g Protein: 6 g Carbs: 17 g

Hot Wings, 4
Cal: 210 Fat: 12 g Protein: 22 g Carbs: 4 g

Mild Wings, 5
Cal: 200 Fat: 12 g Protein: 23 g Carbs: 0 g

ROUND TABLE PIZZA®:

All figures are for 1 slice of thin crust pizza

Cheese
Cal: 160 Fat: 6.2 g Protein: 7 g Carbs: 15 g

Chicken & Garlic Gourmet

260

Low Carb & No Carb Cookbook. (A) 130-Recipes. (B) 85-Low Carb Desserts. (C) 27-Restaurant Guide To Eating Out.

Cal: 170 Fat: 7.2 g Protein: 9 g Carbs: 16 g

Classic Pesto
Cal: 170 Fat: 7.9 g Protein: 7 g Carbs: 16 g

Garden Pesto
Cal: 170 Fat: 7.7 g Protein: 7 g Carbs: 18 g

Gourmet Veggie
Cal: 160 Fat: 6.5 g Protein: 7 g Carbs: 16 g

Guinevere's Garden Delight
Cal: 150 Fat: 5.6 g Protein: 7 g Carbs: 16 g

Maui Zaui w/Red Pizza Sauce
Cal: 170 Fat: 6.5 g Protein: 9 g Carbs: 17 g

Pepperoni
Cal: 170 Fat: 8 g Protein: 8 g Carbs: 15 g

Salute Chicken & Garlic
Cal: 150 Fat: 5.4 g Protein: 8 g Carbs: 16 g

Western BBQ Chicken Supreme
Cal: 170 Fat: 5.6 g Protein: 8 g Carbs: 17 g

RUBY TUESDAY®:

Ruby Tuesday does not provide exact carb counts for all items, but does offer a low carb menu

APPETIZERS –

Chicken Quesadilla
Order with low carb whole wheat tortilla

Spicy Buffalo Wings

261

Low Carb & No Carb Cookbook. (A) 130-Recipes. (B) 85-Low Carb Desserts. (C) 27-Restaurant Guide To Eating Out.

SALADS –

Spring Chicken Salad

New Cajun Chicken Salad

Peppercorn Chicken Caesar

ENTREES –

Low Carb Fajitas (Carbs: 24 g)
Served with low carb whole wheat tortillas

Chopped Steak
Grilled chopped steak served with steamed broccoli and low carb creamy mashed cauliflower.

Grilled Cajun Chicken
Grilled Cajun chicken breast served with steamed broccoli and low carb creamy mashed cauliflower.

Low Carb Catch
Broiled Tilapia, Cajun-seasoned and served with steamed broccoli and low carb creamy mashed
cauliflower.

Church Street Chicken
Grilled chicken with sautéed mushrooms, bacon and melted Swiss cheese. Served with steamed broccoli
and rice pilaf with tomatoes and cheese. Make it low carb by substituting the rice pilaf with low carb creamy mashed cauliflower.

Pepper Blue Steak
Ruby's sirloin with blue cheese crumbles and two low carb sides

Top 10 Sirloins –

262
Low Carb & No Carb Cookbook. (A) 130-Recipes. (B) 85-Low Carb Desserts. (C) 27-Restaurant Guide To Eating Out.

Choose two low carb sides

Ruby's Ribeye (Carbs: 13 g)

Choose two low carb sides

Peppercorn Mushroom Steak

Choose two low carb sides
BURGER WRAPS (order a low carb wrap for the bun)

Black and Blue Burger Wrap (Carbs: 13 g)

Burger in a low carb tortilla with blue cheese, lettuce, tomato, onion, pickles, Dijon mustard

Garlic Mushroom Burger Wrap

Smokehouse Burger

Old English Bacon Cheeseburger

Pepper Jack Bacon Burger

Bacon Cheeseburger

Colossal Burger

Hamburger

Cheeseburger

LOW CARB SIDES –

Steamed Broccoli

Creamy Mashed Cauliflower (Carbs: 7 g)

263
Low Carb & No Carb Cookbook. (A) 130-Recipes. (B) 85-Low Carb Desserts. (C) 27-Restaurant Guide To Eating Out.

Creamy Spinach (Carbs: 9 g)

BBQ Pork Crisps (Carbs: 0 g)

DESSERT –

Atkins Low Carb Cheesecake (Carbs: 6 g) has a crunchy nut crust!

SUBWAY®:

Atkins Friendly Wraps (endorsed by Atkins)

Chicken Bacon Ranch
Calories: 480 Fat: 27 g Carbs: 19 g*

Turkey Bacon Melt
Calories: 430 Fat: 25 g Carbs: 22 g*

* 11 grams Net Carbs or less, and the wrap itself, which is made with wheat gluten, cornstarch, oat, sesame flour and soy protein, has only 5 grams Net Carbs.

Cheese & Egg Omelet
Calories: 240 Fat: 17 g Carbs: 2 g

Bacon & Egg Omelet
Calories: 240 Fat: 17 g Carbs: 2 g

Western & Egg Omelet
Calories: 220 Fat: 14 g Carbs: 4 g

Steak & Egg Omelet
Calories: 250 Fat: 15 g Carbs: 3 g

Ham & Egg Omelet
Calories: 230 Fat: 14 g Carbs: 2 g

264

Low Carb & No Carb Cookbook. (A) 130-Recipes. (B) 85-Low Carb Desserts. (C) 27-Restaurant Guide To Eating Out.

Vegetable & Egg Omelet
Calories: 210 Fat: 14 g Carbs: 4 g

Ham Salad
Cal: 112 Fat: 3 g Protein: 12 g Carbs: 11 g

Roast Beef Salad
Cal: 115 Fat: 3 g Protein: 12 g Carbs: 11 g

Roasted Chicken Breast Salad
Cal: 162 Fat: 4 g Protein: 20 g Carbs: 13 g

Steak & Cheese Salad
Cal: 182 Fat: 8 g Protein: 17 g Carbs: 13 g

Subway Club Salad
Cal: 123 Fat: 3 g Protein: 14 g Carbs: 12 g

Turkey & Ham Salad
Cal: 106 Fat: 2 g Protein: 11 g Carbs: 11 g

Turkey Breast Salad
Cal: 101 Fat: 2 g Protein: 12 g Carbs: 11 g

Light Mayonnaise, 1 tsp
Cal: 18 Fat: 2 g Protein: 0 g Carbs: 0 g

French Dressing, Fat Free, 1 Tbsp.
Cal: 18 Fat: 0 g Protein: 0 g Carbs: 4 g

Italian Dressing, Fat Free, 1 Tbsp.
Cal: 5 Fat: 0 g Protein: 0 g Carbs: 1 g

Ranch, Fat Free Dressing, 1 Tbsp.
Cal: 15 Fat: 0 g Protein: 0 g Carbs: 4 g

265
Low Carb & No Carb Cookbook. (A) 130-Recipes. (B) 85-Low Carb Desserts. (C) 27-Restaurant Guide To Eating Out.

Optional Fixings are all no carb: 2 slices bacon, 2 triangles cheese, Mayonnaise, Olive Oil Blend, Vinegar.
2 tsp of Mustard has 1 g of carbs.

TACO BELL®:

Grilled Chicken Burrito
Cal: 390 Fat: 13 g Protein: 12 g Carbs: 19 g

Grilled Chicken Soft Taco
Cal: 200 Fat: 7 g Protein: 14 g Carbs: 17 g

Grilled Steak Soft Taco
Cal: 200 Fat: 7 g Protein: 19 g Carbs: 14 g

Soft Taco
Cal: 210 Fat: 10 g Protein: 20 g Carbs: 11 g

Steak Gordita Supreme
Cal: 300 Fat: 14 g Protein: 27 g Carbs: 17 g

Taco
Cal: 170 Fat: 10 g Protein: 12 g Carbs: 9 g

Tostada
Cal: 250 Fat: 12 g Protein: 27 g Carbs: 10 g

TGI FRIDAYS®:

Tuscan Spinach Dip
Cal: n/a Fat: n/a Protein: n/a Carbs: 17 g

Buffalo Wings
Cal: n/a Fat: n/a Protein: n/a Carbs: 5 g

New York Strip with Blue Cheese
Cal: n/a Fat: n/a Protein: n/a Carbs: 6 g

266

Low Carb & No Carb Cookbook. (A) 130-Recipes. (B) 85-Low Carb Desserts. (C) 27-Restaurant Guide To Eating Out.

Garlic chicken with mixed vegetables
Cal: n/a Fat: n/a Protein: n/a Carbs: 7 g

Char-grilled salmon fillet
Cal: n/a Fat: n/a Protein: n/a Carbs: 6 g

Tuna salad wraps
Cal: n/a Fat: n/a Protein: n/a Carbs: 14 g

Grilled chicken Caesar salad
Cal: n/a Fat: n/a Protein: n/a Carbs: 9 g

Grilled Chicken with Broccoli
Cal: n/a Fat: n/a Protein: n/a Carbs: 17 g
without grilled peppers: 12 grams of carbs

WENDY'S®:

Option: Order hamburgers & cheeseburgers without the bun.

Chicken Nuggets, 5 pieces
Cal: 230 Fat: 16 g Protein: 11 g Carbs: 11 g

Chicken Nugget, Kid's meal, 4 pieces
Cal: 190 Fat: 13 g Protein: 9 g Carbs: 9 g

Honey Mustard Dipping Sauce
Cal: 130 Fat: 12 g Protein: 0 g Carbs: 6 g

BBQ Dipping Sauce
Cal: 45 Fat: 0 g Protein: 0 g Carbs: 10 g

Sweet n Sour Dipping Sauce
Cal: 50 Fat: 0 g Protein: 0 g Carbs: 11 g

Caesar Side Salad
Cal: 110 Fat: 5 g Protein: 10 g Carbs: 7 g

267

Low Carb & No Carb Cookbook. (A) 130-Recipes. (B) 85-Low Carb Desserts. (C) 27-Restaurant Guide To Eating Out.

Deluxe Garden Salad
Cal: 110 Fat: 6 g Protein: 7 g Carbs: 9 g

Grilled Chicken Salad
Cal: 200 Fat: 8 g Protein: 25 g Carbs: 9 g

Side Salad
Cal: 60 Fat: 3 g Protein: 4g Carbs: 5 g

French, Fat Free Dressing, 2 Tbsp.
Cal: 35 Fat: 0 g Protein: 0 g Carbs: 8 g

French Dressing, 2 Tbsp.
Cal: 120 Fat: 10 g Protein: 0 g Carbs: 6 g

Italian Caesar Dressing, 2 Tbsp.
Cal: 150 Fat: 16 g Protein: 0 g Carbs: 2 g

Ranch, 2 Tbsp.
Cal: 100 Fat: 10 g Protein: 0 g Carbs: 1 g

****

I thank you so much for purchasing the: **Low Carb & No Carb Cookbook with 130-Recipes, 85-Low Carb Desserts and 27-Restaurant Guide To Eating Out.

268
Low Carb & No Carb Cookbook. (A) 130-Recipes. (B) 85-Low Carb Desserts. (C) 27-Restaurant Guide To Eating Out.

**Please return and leave a review about your experience. Thank you and have a fantastic day.

-Best Wishes.

Sincerely,

Andrew Bennett.

****

Made in the USA
Coppell, TX
18 December 2022